It's Not Rocket Science

A real diet for the real world

By Anne Elliott

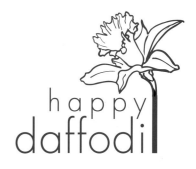

happy
daffodil

Published by Happy Daffodil
556 Finchley Road, London NW11 8DD

First Edition 2006

ISBN   0-9552911-0-0
       978-0-9552911-0-4

A CIP catalogue record for this book is available from the
British Library.

Note

Every effort has been made to ensure the contents of this book, which have been obtained from reliable sources,
are technically correct and accurate as at the date of this publication. To the fullest extent permitted by law, the
author and the publisher do not make any (and expressly disclaims all) representations or warranties of any kind
with respect to the contents and disclaim any liability for any responsibility for loss, damage or personal injury
arising as a result of the contents of this book. The contents are in no way intended to replace professional
medical care or advice from a qualified practitioner. The contents of this book cannot and should not be used as
a basis for diagnosis or choice of treatment. If you have any concerns about your health you should consult a
doctor immediately.

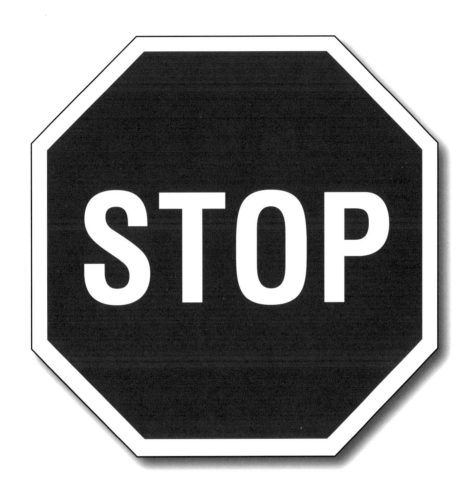

PLEASE NOTE THAT BEFORE UNDERTAKING ANY
FORM OF DIET OR EXERCISE REGIME IT IS
RECOMMENDED THAT YOU CONSULT WITH A DOCTOR
OR QUALIFIED PRACTITIONER.

This is YOUR reference book. To make it personal and pertinent to you, I hope you'll make notes wherever you need them. And don't forget to fill in the sections with the ✏️ symbol!

Age isn't important unless you're a cheese. — Anon

WHAT THIS BOOK <u>CAN'T</u> DO

1. It can't turn you into Jennifer Lopez/Brad Pitt
2. It can't get you into that itzy bitzy bikini in 2 weeks
3. It can't make your life perfect
4. It can't bring about world peace

WHAT THIS BOOK <u>CAN</u> DO

1. It can help you look the best you've ever been
2. It can show you how to have more energy
3. It can help you feel great about yourself
4. It can help you find the confidence to go for goals you thought were out of your reach
5. It can help you get into the clothes you've always wanted to
6. It can show you how to be fit and healthy
7. It can get you out of the section of the population considered obese if you're one of them
8. It can show you how to safeguard the health and fitness of your children

DO YOU NEED THIS BOOK?

Read through the next few pages to find out.

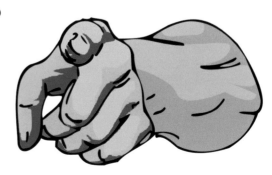

HERE ARE 4 METHODS YOU CAN USE

1. BMI — WHAT IS IT ?

Body Mass Index (BMI) is a standardised way to work out if you are a healthy weight for your height, allowing for normal differences in build and frame size. If you are a body builder or athlete, it will not work, because you will have more heavy muscle. Nor does it work for children, who are still growing. But for most of us it's a good guide. To work out your BMI, you'll need to know your weight and height.

HOW TO WORK OUT YOUR BMI

It's a simple calculation which can be worked out using either metric or imperial measures.

METRIC: $$\frac{\textbf{Your Weight in kilograms}}{\textbf{Height in metres x Height in metres}}$$

For example: my weight today is 68kg, my height is 1.78m

$$\frac{68}{1.78 \times 1.78} = 21.5$$

IMPERIAL: $$\frac{\textbf{Your Weight in pounds (lbs)}}{\textbf{Height in inches x Height in inches}} \times \textbf{703}$$

For example: my weight today is 10st 10lbs (150lbs), my height is 5ft10 (70in)

$$\frac{150}{70 \times 70} \times 703 = 21.5$$

My BMI = 21.5. We then check our BMI against the table below.

BMI	CLASSIFICATION
Less than 18.4	Underweight
18.5–24.9	Healthy
25–29.9	Overweight
30–34.9	Obese (class 1)
35–39.9	Obese (class 2)
Over 40	Morbidly or severely obese

source: www.nhsdirect.nhs.uk

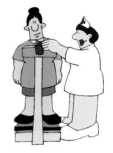

Image from clipartheaven.com

NOW ITS YOUR TURN.

My Height is:

My Weight is:

METRIC: $\dfrac{\text{Your weight in kilograms}}{\text{Height in metres} \times \text{Height in metres}}$ =

IMPERIAL: $\dfrac{\text{Your weight in pounds (lbs)}}{\text{Height in inches} \times \text{Height in inches}}$ x 703 =

YOUR BMI IS:

2. WHAT IS IDEAL WEIGHT?

Find out how much you should weigh by looking at the charts below. This chart is in stones and kilograms. For pounds, please see the table on page 6.

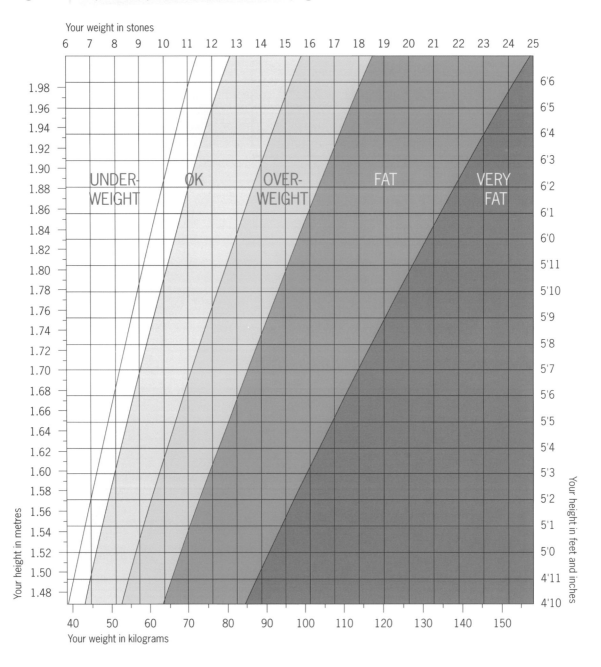

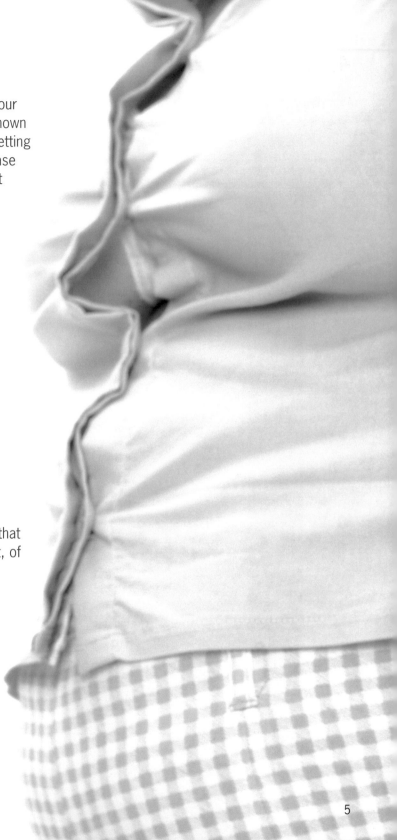

3. A BIG TUM!

The amount of fat deposited around your waist, stomach and chest has been shown to be a big factor in your chance of getting diseases such as cardiovascular disease and type 2 diabetes. Check your waist measurement. It doesn't matter what your height or weight are for this.

MEN
Substantial risk of disease
= more than 40 inches (102cm)

WOMEN
Substantial risk of disease
= more than 35 inches (88cm)

There's food for thought.

Something else to chew on:

The World Health Organisation states that globally 1 billion adults are overweight, of which 300 million are obese.

source: World Health Organisation

4. HEIGHT VS. WEIGHT

For kilograms, stones and metres please see the graph on page 6.

Height	Ideal Body Weight	
	Male	Female
4'10"	85–103lbs	81–99lbs
4'11"	90–110lbs	86–105lbs
5'0"	95–117lbs	90–110lbs
5'1"	101–123lbs	95–116lbs
5'2"	106–130lbs	99–121lbs
5'3"	112–136lbs	104–127lbs
5'4"	117–143lbs	108–132lbs
5'5"	122–150lbs	113–138lbs
5'6"	128–156lbs	117–143lbs
5'7"	133–163lbs	122–149lbs
5'8"	139–169lbs	126–154lbs
5'9"	144–176lbs	131–160lbs
5'10"	149–183lbs	135–165lbs
5'11"	155–189lbs	140–171lbs
6'0"	160–196lbs	144–176lbs
6'1"	166–202lbs	149–182lbs
6'2"	171–209lbs	153–187lbs
6'3"	176–216lbs	158–193lbs
6'4"	182–222lbs	162–198lbs
6'5"	187–229lbs	167–204lbs
6'6"	193–235lbs	171–209lbs

SO WHY THIS BOOK IN PARTICULAR?

This is a no-nonsense, straightforward, practical approach to losing weight and getting fit. It is for all of us; people with busy lives with the usual sprinkling of problems. As you can see below, I developed this programme the hard way! Other diets had failed for me, so I had to find a way that fitted my life as a working woman, mother, wife, housekeeper and everything else I do in the bits in between and don't forget that I love FOOD. This book is the result of my search. It's how I lost weight. It's a real diet, for real people living real lives. I hope it suits you too.

BEFORE

AFTER

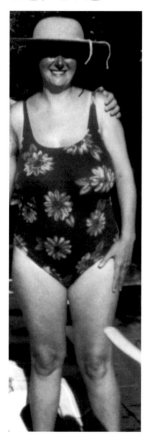

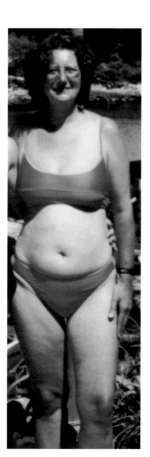

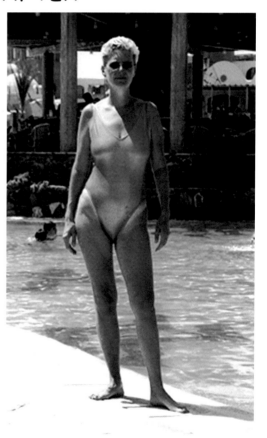

1999

2000

2002

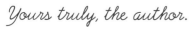

Yours truly, the author.

WHY <u>ME</u>?

So many people asked me how I'd done it. Friends who did not see me for long periods of time were amazed by the improvements not only in my looks but also in my energy and positive approach to life. It has made me look and feel 15 years younger. I'd never done any exercise before I started this diet. I'm not a scientist or dietician, I'm not a fitness fanatic. I'm just a middle aged woman who had tried most of the other diets and failed—a big yo-yo dieter—who felt worn down by the stresses of life. I couldn't bare to look in the mirror at myself because all I saw was a fat, unfit, tired woman who had eaten her way through 2 pregnancies, wore tents of different descriptions and had no future hope of improvement.

I was visiting my sister one day who was also struggling with her weight. She was moaning as we all do, "How ever hard I try, I can't lose weight?" At that moment her man walked through the kitchen and rather bluntly said to us both, "It's not rocket science—just eat less and do more exercise." EUREKA! The light bulb switched on in my head. My God, that's it! It is that simple. If I do nothing more than that I will lose weight. So from that simple start I began a journey of self-discovery to find the me inside the fat lump. I found out a lot out about my motivations and how I tick and about how to look after myself properly and eat well. I lost a lot of weight and from spending my whole life trying to avoid exercise, I got fit, then I got super fit then I took up boxing and began to love using this body I'd found. It's been a wonderful journey.

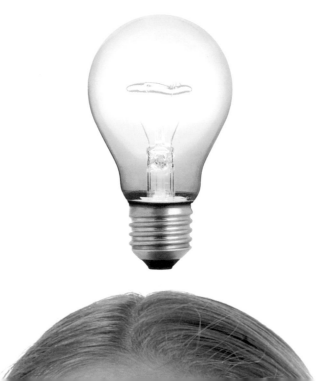

WHY <u>YOU</u>?

I ask you to take your own journey. You never know, you may be just what the world of freestyle skateboarding has been waiting for. Or perhaps its time to see how good you really look in a size 10 Prada suit.

Why not have an outrageously wild challenge. How about saying to yourself, 'In 2 years I'm going to run the London Marathon for charity.' Does that sound ridiculous? Don't laugh. If someone had said to me in 1999 (just look at my photo on page 7) 'In 2 years you will get in a boxing ring with an amateur champion for a 3 round charity exhibition.' I would have thought you were insane! But I did it.

This book will take you through stage-by-stage the goods and bads of trying to lose weight.

PLEASE DON'T GO STRAIGHT TO THE DIET PAGES. YOU NEED TO ANSWER ALL THE QUESTIONS IN THE FIRST PART BEFORE YOU START TO DIET.

Please write in the book as much as you need. Add your thoughts along the way, answer all the questions, take as much time as you need. This is not a prescriptive 'one way' only method as we are all very different and have had different experiences to get us where we are now. The fail-safe method of success here is BE HONEST WITH YOURSELF. The more honest you can be about your own strengths and weaknesses, which will become apparent as you work through the book, the more successful you will be.

I have avoided long technical essays but have tried to keep things short and to the point. For the scientists amongst you, forgive me as I have tried to explain in general terms the principles of losing weight. I know there are many exceptions dependent on specific circumstances and for those of you who develop an irresistible urge to find out more about calorific values or major muscle groups or any aspect of nutrition and fitness I have enclosed a book list for you to discover more.

Don't be under any illusion—this diet is not magic. It's not an overnight cure. It's not even controversial. Miracle cures don't exist. I think that's one of the reasons we all fail time after time. We chase the dream that people offer—(If you eat nothing but radishes for 6 months, you'll lose 28 stone (177.8kg/392lbs) and be rich and successful beyond your wildest dreams) I've probably even tried it. Don't tell me, you did too!

This diet will take determination on your part when times get tough or life throws something unexpected at you and you reach for a chocolate bar. It may well be the hardest thing you ever do. You will need to ditch the excuses once and for all. Why not take the occasional photo of yourself like I did. It does you good to look back (See inside back cover). That fatter you will feel more and more like a stranger, both physically and mentally. It also reminds you why you are doing this.

I hope your personal journey, whatever it may entail, will be as rewarding as mine has been. So with your pen in hand, (and as the Chinese say, the longest journey starts with one step), lets begin with finding out why we failed before so that we can make sure we don't make the same mistakes twice.

Be healthy and prosper.

Good luck.

notes

I've been on a diet for two weeks and all I've lost is two weeks.
— Totie Fields

WHY DID I FAIL BEFORE? ☹

Many of the popular diets around are very successful and suit certain people. If you are one of them then good for you, stick with it. However, if like me you have tried most of them and failed, it is imperative to ask yourself why. Consider if a particular diet lasted longer than the others and what was it that gave it the edge for you. There may be something in there you could use again. Think about each 'type' of diet you have tried and think about what was wrong about it for you and if anything in it worked.

Here is my personal list of failure reasons:

1. I LOVE FOOD. Anywhere, anytime, any kind.

2. Calorie counting diets were just too obsessive. I spent hours reading packaging and although I was allowed that piece of chocolate cake, it made me want more.

3. Starvation and extreme diets such as the cabbage diet made me feel ill and all the weight piled back on as soon as the 'week' was over.

4. Restricted food diets such as the egg diet just made me loathe eggs by day 4, even though I quite like eggs.

5. High fat–no carbohydrate diet—no good for me. I love bread, pasta and cheese.

6. Doing exercise was minus 523 on my priority list of things to do.

7. Low fat diet was for me the most successful but eventually failed because I pined for a cheese butty or crumpets with lashings of butter.

My own conclusions:

1. It was pointless me spending time on any diet that stopped me having foods I loved.

2. I did learn that I was quite happy filling up on more vegetables and fruit if I had to.

3. The one big thing I was missing was exercise.

Now it's your turn. Remember, be honest with yourself. It may take some time for you to mull the question over. Don't worry. You can always come back to it as things occur later to you.

Today is the tomorrow we worried about yesterday. — Anon

WHY DID <u>YOU</u> FAIL BEFORE?

I failed before because:

1.
2.
3.
4.
5.
6.
7.
8.

My conclusions are:

1.
2.
3.
4.
5.

I can resist anything but temptation
— Oscar Wilde

✳ BE HONEST! ✳

WHICH ONE HAVE YOU USED?

So now you have a clearer idea about **why** you failed in the past, what about the present? Do any of these excuses ring true with you now?

"What's the point? The last diet I did I lost 2 stone but I've put it all back on plus some."

Good for you. You did it before which means you can do it again. But this time I want you to understand how and why you lost the weight so that you can keep it off. When people diet without doing any exercise the body uses the fat stores that you want it to, but also takes away some lean muscle. When you go back to your old eating habits you put back on the fat but not the muscle. Thus your weight goes up. If you have yo-yo dieted this will have happened time after time. The good news is that it doesn't have to be like this. Read on.

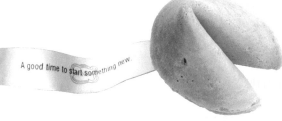

A good time to start something new

"What do you mean, 'do more exercise'? I'm on the go all day; cleaning the house, looking after the children, going to work. I'm on my feet from the moment I get up."

I've used this one myself. Any time I got at the end of the day, I was so exhausted all I could do was veg in front of the tele. Funnily enough, even though I found 2–3 hours to do nothing each day, I just felt more and more tired as time went on.

The body has an amazing ability to adapt to what you demand of it, and although you may be on your feet all day, this is not exercise. This is normal for 'your' body. In order to get fitter, you must do something that either raises your heart rate a little or make it work against resistance (weights). You have to push your body to do more than it would do in a normal day. If you saw the recent series 'I'm a celebrity—get me out of here' the

participants were forced to live in a much more physically demanding situation than they were used to, with less food to eat. It hurt them all for the first few days, but gradually their bodies adapted to the demands of their surroundings. They all came out leaner and fitter. I am not saying that we have to move en mass to the nearest jungle and give ourselves a bad time, but we have to fight against our natural inclinations to eat as much as possible and to do only what we can get away with. Finally, considers builders. They have one of the most physically demanding jobs around. Are they all fit, lean and perfect examples of health? I don't think so. Their bodies adapt to the strenuous, daily, job requirements. They still put on weight.

I'm at an age when my back goes out more than I do.
— Phyllis Diller

"I don't know why I'm putting on so much weight. I hardly eat a thing."

Section 4 'Where are you today?' will soon put paid to this one.

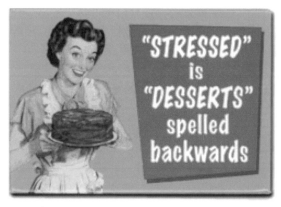

Magnet from funkyfridge.com

14

" I just can't stick to diets. After a week or two I fall off the rails. Something always happens that sends me back to comfort eating."

This is where old-fashioned dogged determination is the only answer. You have to make sure you want to lose weight, have good reasons for doing so and take responsibility for what you put in your mouth. Life is always going to throw problems your way. You can't waste your time blaming everyone and everything else for your weight issues. Don't comfort eat. The problems don't go away—especially your weight problem. You need to find another way. Gosh, that sounds a bit hard. But perhaps if nothing else has helped it might be time to look this one in the eye and face it off in your own way. If you use food to help with more deep seated emotional issues please read page 52 "Take control of you."

" I'm always dieting because I know there's a J-Lo/Brad Pitt in there somewhere if I could only get down to her/him."

A problem we all face is the relentless bombardment of images of 'beautiful' women and men. But we all have to get real here. Unfortunately, the genetic dice is not fair and no amount of dieting and beauty treatments are going to turn me into Jennifer Aniston. But I can be the best 'me' possible. If you feel good about yourself and the way you look you will find a confidence that attracts others.

"I have no time in the day to exercise."

If someone said to you 'I will give you £100 a week if you walk round the park for 20 minutes a day', I bet you would find the time then. It's not finding the time that's the problem; it's finding the reason. So how about if you exercise for 20 minutes a day in 3 months you will be in 2 dress sizes smaller, or you'll be able to run and kick a ball round and enjoy it, just like you did when you were young. Find your own reason. You can also look at ways of exercising during the day that are not formal sports.

I'm tired of all this nonsense about beauty being only skin deep. That's deep enough. What do you want, an adorable pancreas?
— Jean Kerr

"I can't attempt this diet because I smoke."

So what's that got to do with anything? You don't need me to tell you how bad smoking is for you, but it certainly won't get in the way of eating less. As far as doing exercise is concerned it won't stop you doing that either, however, it does give you a bit of a handicap. But IT DOESN'T STOP YOU DOING IT! I speak from experience. When I began losing weight I was a 20 a day girl. It just took me longer to get fit and I wheezed a lot more. I naturally began cutting down, as I got fitter. Eventually, I had to make a decision. I couldn't box and smoke. Incompatible. I wanted to be able to stay in the ring for 4 rounds so after a few attempts I managed to stop smoking. I found my reason to stop.

Your weight problem and your smoking problem are 2 different problems. Aim for slow steady improvements with both and make each improvement last rather than rushing at everything and failing. Why not ask your GP for extra help with quitting smoking. There may be locally based support groups you could consider. If you feel you have the strength of mind to do the whole lot alone then I wish you every success, but remember, it's not failure to ask for help.

"I'm prone to be fat, I can't help it. I'm sure it's my thyroid, bowels, stomach, blah, blah, blah."

OK, there are a small number of people who do have a specific medical problem that hinders their metabolism and weight control. The problem most of us have is in our mind and we look for excuses not to deal with it. If you believe you really do have a physical problem for your weight problem then SEE A DOCTOR IMMEDIATELY and find out how to deal with it medically and safely. If your doctor says you are perfectly all right, then you have to take control of the problem in your mind and deal with it.

"I haven't got time or inclination to cook complicated meals."

Eating healthily does not mean spending hours peeling grapes, or producing a perfect Moule Marinere or spending the whole weekly food budget on Japanese rice grown on the southern slopes of Mount Fuji. This will be explained later in the book.

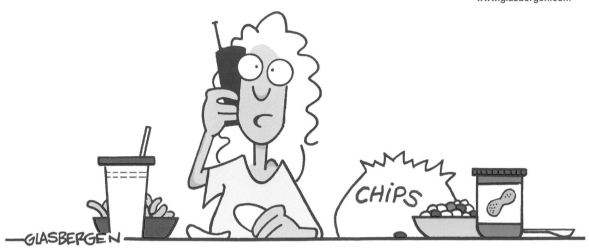

"I'm on a low-carb diet.
Whenever I feel low, I eat carbs!"

"It's personality that matters more than what lies within."

And what may lie within a severely overweight person? A heart that is straining at the edges to do its job, a liver that can't process all the rubbish that is thrown its way, lungs that have trouble getting enough air in to walk up some stairs, joints that are under strain from carrying too much body weight: heart disease, diabetes, and a myriad of other unpleasant, unnecessary ailments round the corner waiting to pounce. Have you ever seen the self confidence of someone who has lost a lot of weight and feels good about themselves? Big personality boost.

"The children won't eat proper food and I can't afford to waste it."

I understand this. It's very easy for kids to get into bad eating habits. The pressure on them to eat junk is even greater than on us. You will have World War III on your hands if you try to change them overnight. A slower approach can be taken where foods are introduced bit by bit until they become normal. Also it's up to you to set a good example. If the norm in your house is to eat well-balanced, good food, they are more likely to take that into their adult lives.

Please write down your current excuses:

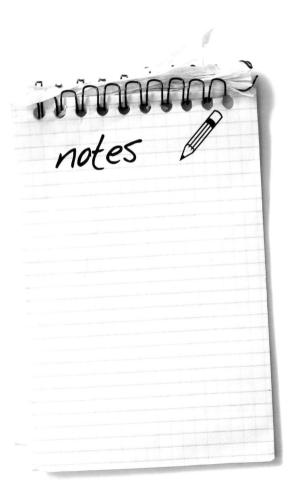

We are indeed much more than what we eat, but what we eat can nevertheless help us to be much more than what we are.
— Adelle Davis

WHERE ARE YOU TODAY?

Now we've recognised past failures and present excuses for not doing anything, let's look at the present under a microscope. Before you can change your eating habits you have to know exactly what they are. Therefore, for the next 4 days please fill in the food chart. You must write down absolutely everything that passes your lips from the moment you get up till you go to bed.

This includes all drinks and any extras like sugars in hot drinks or cereal, or salt on food. Try to be as specific about amounts as you can without having to weigh everything, i.e. if your dinner is piled like a mountain then it's likely you have given yourself large portions. If you've got an inch thick of butter and jam on your toast, make a note of it. Be careful if you 'nibble' while you are preparing food or if you finish off the children's leftovers. It all counts. If it goes past your lips—it gets written down.

EAT AS YOU NORMALLY WOULD WHILST YOU ARE FILLING IN THE CHART.

I think you will be shocked by the amount you are putting away. If you truly are eating like a mouse and yet piling on the weight, take the food chart to your doctor and find out if there is a medical reason behind it.

If you are eating a well balanced diet in reasonable amounts, it may be that what is missing is the exercise.

If you are eating too much or the wrong kinds of things then carry on with us to learn how to improve matters.

Please use this monthly planner page to help you with your diet preparation.

Last Month 30	31	This Month 1	2	3	4	5
6	7	8	9	10	11	12
13	14	15	16	17	18	19
20	21	22	23	24	25	26
27	28	29	30	Next Month 1	2	3

I drive too fast to worry about cholesterol. — Anon

DAY 1	DATE		
TIME	WHAT I ATE/DRANK	AMOUNT	EXTRAS

END OF DAY

How many different fruit and veg did you eat?

How many processed foods did you eat?

How many things had sugar in them?   none / few / lots

How many things had salt in them?   none / few / lots

How many things had fat in them?   none / few / lots

How many glasses of water did you drink?

A chocolate mousse you didn't order has no calories, therefore, get your friend to order desert and you taste half of it! — Anon

DAY 2	DATE		
TIME	WHAT I ATE/DRANK	AMOUNT	EXTRAS

END OF DAY

How many different fruit and veg did you eat?

How many processed foods did you eat?

How many things had sugar in them?   none / few / lots

How many things had salt in them?   none / few / lots

How many things had fat in them?   none / few / lots

How many glasses of water did you drink?

Children's views of the human body:

A molecule is so small it cannot be seen by the naked observer.
Blood flows down one leg and up the other one.
The alimentary canal is located in the north of India.

DAY 3	DATE		
TIME	WHAT I ATE/DRANK	AMOUNT	EXTRAS

END OF DAY
How many different fruit and veg did you eat?
How many processed foods did you eat?
How many things had sugar in them?   none / few / lots
How many things had salt in them?   none / few / lots
How many things had fat in them?   none / few / lots
How many glasses of water did you drink?

The best part of beauty is that which no picture can express.
— Francis Bacon

DAY 4	DATE		
TIME	WHAT I ATE/DRANK	AMOUNT	EXTRAS

END OF DAY

How many different fruit and veg did you eat?

How many processed foods did you eat?

How many things had sugar in them?   none / few / lots

How many things had salt in them?   none / few / lots

How many things had fat in them?   none / few / lots

How many glasses of water did you drink?

Age is bad, but consider the alternative. — Anon

SO HOW DID YOU DO?

What became glaringly obvious?

Are you single-handedly keeping the soft drink industry afloat?

Did you have the minimum recommended 5 different types of fruit and vegetables per day?

Did you remember to include the sugar, fat and salt that is put in processed foods'
— just look on the packet.

Do you eat a wide variety of foods?

Do you eat a good balance of fruit, vegetables, grains (bread etc), carbohydrate, and protein?

Do you snack on crisps, sweets, chocolate?

Do you live on potatoes?

How do you feel about what you have eaten over the last 4 days?

      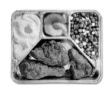

Magnets from funkyfridge.com

What can you conclude from your food chart? Firstly the bad points then the good points. Make it as long or a short as you need. The conclusions will give you informed information about your existing strengths that you can use and weaknesses that you can now alter.

MY EXISTING BAD POINTS ARE:
i.e. I eat too much processed food.

1.

2.

3.

4.

5.

6.

7.

8.

9.

10.

MY EXISTING GOOD POINTS ARE:
i.e. I eat 4 kinds of fruit and veg a day, which I could easily push up to 5.

1.

2.

3.

4.

5.

6.

7.

8.

9.

10.

Order is the shape upon which beauty depends. — Pearl Buck

A LITTLE KNOWLEDGE CAN GO A LONG WAY

You should now have a better idea of what you're up against, but before we can begin the diet in earnest, there are a few things that are imperative to understand so that you can have more control over your eating habits. I have kept it as simple and as general as possible and I do apologise if you already know this information, but it does no harm to refresh your memory occasionally and I am assuming that like me, you may not have a scientific background.

PLEASE DON'T SKIP THIS BIT.

It is central to understanding the diet and being able to maintain a healthy eating regime after you have finished.

We need to look at food and your body. How and why it works. If you understand the principle of what is happening every time you put food in your mouth, you have the knowledge to control food as opposed to food controlling you. I did say that this is not a calorie counting diet and it's not. But it is important to understand how the body processes food and the easiest way to see how the body does that is to understand the humble calorie.

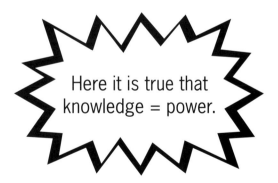

Here it is true that knowledge = power.

27

EAT TO LIVE OR LIVE TO EAT

All cars need fuel to go, from the grandest
BMW to the most clapped out banger.
The faster they go, the more fuel they eat up.

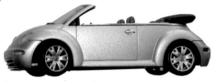

Photographer: Sencer Saygiver

We also need fuel to move. The more we move, the more fuel we need. But unlike the car, which stops using fuel when you turn it off, we never turn off. Even when we're not moving, say being a couch potato, we still need a little fuel to keep the heart pumping or your eyelids blinking or to help your thumb push the button on the remote to change channels. The body is an amazing thing. There are hundreds of movements happening without you being aware of them, just keeping you alive and kicking.

Food is our fuel and we have a wide selection to pick from. All foods have a caloric value but what is a calorie?

A calorie is a measured unit of energy (in this case heat)

Just like we can measure length in centimetres, it doesn't matter if we're measuring the length of a book, which may be 21cm, or a long wall which may be 5034cm, the value of a centimetre is the same.

Well so it is with a calorie. The value of a calorie is the same when you are trying to measure 2 different foods. For example, lets look at the energy stored in an apple compared to a lump of chocolate. In order to compare them, we have to make sure that the weight of both is the same:

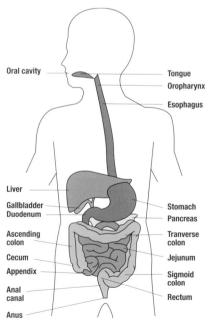

100g (3.5oz) of chocolate = 505 kcal
100g (3.5oz) of apple   = 52 kcal

We can see from this that chocolate has more energy packed into it, and if we wanted a quick snack to fill our stomach and not have hunger pains, then the apple would be a better bet, as we could eat 10 times more apple than chocolate to get the same amount of calories. Whereas, if we ate the chocolate, we'd still need more food to fill our stomach because it's not bulky enough to make us feel full. 10 apples would certainly fill me up whereas a few squares of chocolate definitely wouldn't. I know you actually wouldn't want to eat 10 apples in one go, but you see what I mean.

We can easily see how many calories are in other food, especially if the food is sold in a packet or tin.

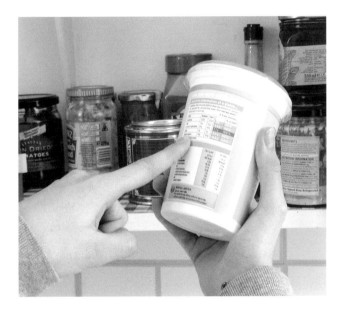
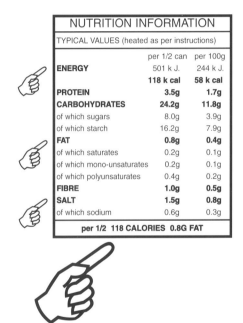

NUTRITION INFORMATION

TYPICAL VALUES (heated as per instructions)

	per 1/2 can	per 100g
ENERGY	501 k J.	244 k J.
	118 k cal	**58 k cal**
PROTEIN	**3.5g**	**1.7g**
CARBOHYDRATES	**24.2g**	**11.8g**
of which sugars	8.0g	3.9g
of which starch	16.2g	7.9g
FAT	**0.8g**	**0.4g**
of which saturates	0.2g	0.1g
of which mono-unsaturates	0.2g	0.1g
of which polyunsaturates	0.4g	0.2g
FIBRE	**1.0g**	**0.5g**
SALT	**1.5g**	**0.8g**
of which sodium	0.6g	0.3g

per 1/2 118 CALORIES 0.8G FAT

If you look on the side of a packet or tin you have in your kitchen you will see a list of all the ingredients and their nutritional values. In Great Britain, manufacturers must put this information on by law. On this, you can find the caloric value for the food inside per 100g (3.5oz) and per serving. It is normally the top item on the list.

	Per serving	Per 100g (3.5oz)	
ENERGY	60kj	161kj	kj – ignore this one – different system
	14kcal	**384kcal**	**kcal – this is the one we want**

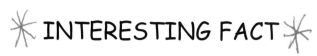

INTERESTING FACT

In the same way that we can measure temperature in celsius or fahrenheit or length in inches or centimetres, heat energy can be measured in kilocalories (kcal) or kilojoules (kj). 1kcal = approximately 4kj. Kj is the more modern system but we still seem to like our kcals. This list can be useful, especially if the food is processed and has a lot of ingredients. They have done the hard work for you and worked out the caloric value of all the ingredients together. Have a look for yourself. You would be amazed at the amount of kcals you find in processed food compared to something simpler. Compare a tin of tomatoes to a meat pie or a pre-prepared meal you might have in the freezer. This is because processed foods tend to have a lot of fat and sugar in them which both have a high calorific value. The bad news is that it's more than likely all the foods you love to eat tend to have a high caloric value.

Look for yourself.

Take 5 items you already have in your kitchen, that you eat on a regular basis and find out what's in them. I have made some suggestions, but please feel free to choose your own.

ITEM	kcal per serving	kcal per 100g (3.5oz)
1. Tin of tomatoes		
2. Packet of crisps		
3. Breakfast cereal		
4. Ready meal		
5. Oven chips		

Or your choices:

ITEM	kcal per serving	kcal per 100g (3.5oz)
1.		
2.		
3.		
4.		
5.		

The recommended amount of calories needed by an average female is 2000kcal per day and 2500 kcal for men to maintain average body weight. That means for a woman everything you eat and drink in a day should add up to 2000kcal.

In order to lose weight steadily and slowly that number should be:

1250 for women who want to lose less than 1st (6.4kg/14lbs) — 1500 for men

1500 for women who want to lose 1st to 3st (6.4kg/14lbs to 19kg/42lbs) — 1750 for men

1750 for women who want to lose more than 3st (19kg/42lbs) — 2000 for men

---

You want to aim at losing 2–3lbs (0.9–1.4kg) per week.

 INTERESTING FACT

Much of the energy we use is simply needed to maintain our body temperature at 37°C (98.6°F). If you decided to take a hearty walk in the Arctic, you would need 5000–8000kcal per day.

We now have an idea of how to find out the relative values of the food we eat, but so what, I hear you say.

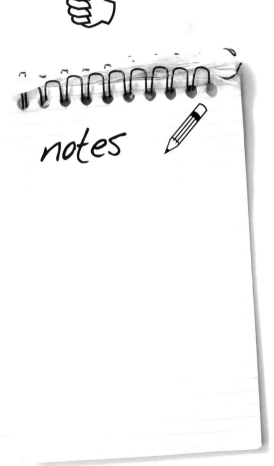

Ask not what you can do for your country. Ask what's for lunch.
— Orson Welles

ALL CHANGE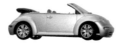

Let us think about the car again. In order to travel the 200 miles (322km) to see my mother, I know I must put in 7.5 gallons (34 litres) of petrol. The car takes the petrol and converts it into movement. I know I roughly need 7.5 gallons (34 litres) because 0.26 gallons (1 litre) will take me about 6 miles (9.65km).

The petrol (litres) is changed into movement (miles/km). So it is with us with food and movement, but you'll never guess what, it's easier with us because we use calories to measure the amount of potential energy in a food as well as the energy used to do something, like this:

1 apple (52kcal) = 15 minutes cleaning the house (52kcal)
1 large chocolate chip cookie (80kcal) = 10 minutes digging the garden (80kcal)
1 pack cheese and onion crisps (130kcal) = 20 minutes very brisk walk (130kcal)

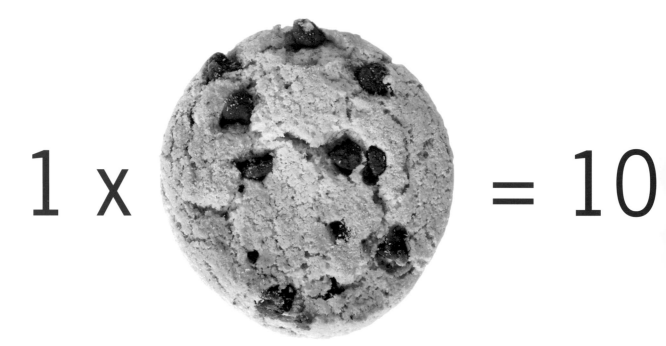

1 x ⬤ = 10

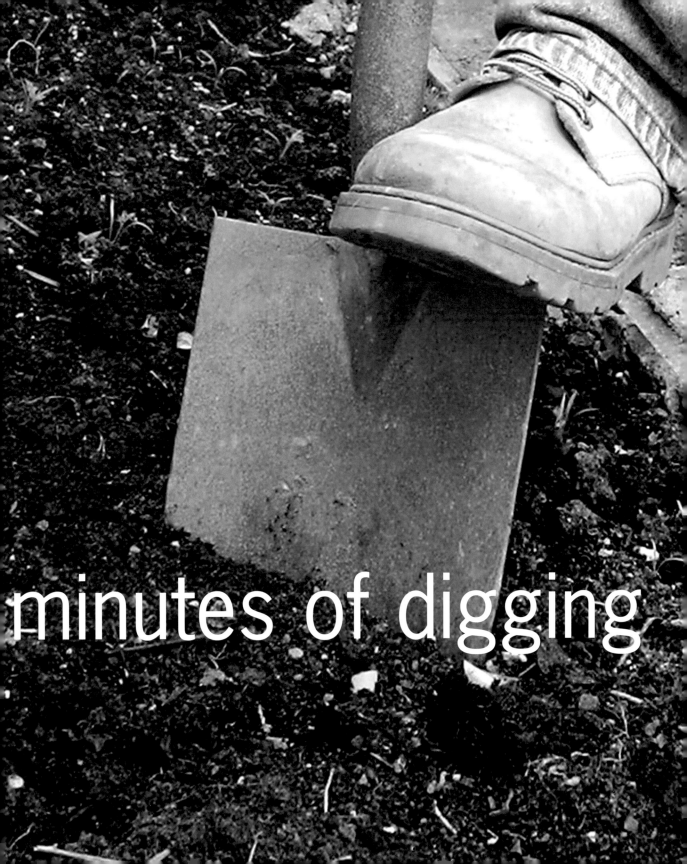

minutes of digging

Never eat more than you can lift. — Miss Piggy

THE BIG IDEA

When we eat, our bodies turn food into energy that we can use up how and when we want.

The word 'energy' is the key. The food contains potential energy and the body uses that energy to move.

Our bodies work most efficiently when they are constantly topped up with food throughout the day.

All the food we eat can be given a caloric value.

All the movement we do in a day can be given a caloric value.

So, in a day we could count up all the calories we have burnt off doing activities and keeping our bodies ticking over and compare the total to how many we have eaten.

Its like a weighing scale—calories in vs. calories out

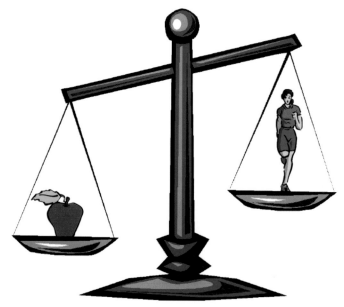

CALORIES IN   CALORIES OUT
Food we have eaten   VS.   Activity we have done

WHY AM I OVERWEIGHT?

For those of you who would like to find out how the body uses food in more detail, I have included a book list for further reading but for everyone, here is the general principle.

If you have eaten 2000kcal and burnt off 2000kcal in a day your weight will stay the same. No problem.

If you have eaten 2000kcal and burnt off 2500kcal in a day you will lose weight.

If you have eaten 2000kcal and burnt off 1500kcal in a day you will put weight on.

But what happens when you eat 2000 kcal but only use 1990? There are 10 left unused. Not many to worry about. But what if that keeps happening day on day, week on week, month on month? It becomes a lot of unused energy.

The body's answer is to store those unused calories and unused energy as fat for a rainy day. We are all still deep down cavemen and our body thinks, 'there may be no food around tomorrow'. If there is no food around it can go back to its storehouse and change the fat back to energy. So it converts the unwanted energy into fat and tucks it away around the body, the obvious being under the skin where you can see it, but also less obviously around vital organs. Trouble is that in many of us the body's storehouse has become a jumbo-sized warehouse with fat stored in every nook and cranny.

THAT IS WHY YOU ARE OVERWEIGHT

So if you are prepared to train at the level of a world class athlete you could carry on eating the same amount as you do now plus some, because you would be burning off more than you are putting in. If you're not ready to do that you have to reduce your intake of food and up your amount of exercise. It really is that straightforward.

FAT IS UNUSED ENERGY

...nc is a great teacher, but unfortunately it kills all its pupils.
— Berlioz

THE SPEEDOMETER

We all know someone who is stick thin and however much they eat, never puts on an ounce of weight. Don't you just hate them, especially if you go up a dress size just by looking at a piece of Gateaux? How do they do it? We're back to our genetic dice. They probably have a naturally high metabolic rate.

Metabolism or the metabolic rate is the speed at which the body converts food to energy. So people who have a high metabolic rate can tap into the available energy quickly and burn it off. If you have a high metabolic rate you tend to be a more energetic person. Have you ever noticed how small children have this constant need to keep moving to get rid of the excess energy they feel.

Sadly, as we get older it slows down. Most people, by the time they're 40 say 'I don't have anywhere near the energy I used to have when I was 20'. As we age our activity levels go down, our metabolism slows and yet our food intake stays the same or increases. Hence weight gain, loss of energy and, what's worse, we lose the will to fight against it.

A VIRTUOUS CIRCLE

Your metabolism can be speeded up by doing exercise on a regular basis. As your muscles become toned, stronger and more used, you will need more energy to maintain them and your metabolic rate will increase to supply the extra need—it's common sense really. This also means you burn calories quicker than before, even during resting (RMR - resting metabolic rate).

If you try and diet without the exercising, approximately 25% of the weight you lose will be lean muscle. So...

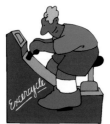 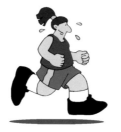 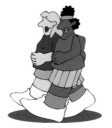 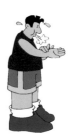

Images from clipartheaven.com

...as long as you are exercising your muscles regularly and your calorie intake is lessened, your body will look to the fat stored for the shortfall rather than the muscle and you will lose weight, have a great shape and have more energy to do more exercise which means your metabolism rises and burns calories quicker which means you lose more weight and have more energy to do more exercise...

training

more energy

faster maetabolism

more calories burned

I found that once I got this circle turning, I was doing more exercise so I needed more and more good food to support it. I was eating a lot. But this was because my body needed the extra energy for all the demands I was putting on it. I also knew it was OK because I was burning it off. It's a great feeling to have that you can eat as much as you want and still be losing weight!

A friend of mine told me that she also noticed that as she got fitter, she found she wanted to eat good food rather than rubbish. Her body knew what it needed to perform. She just started listening to it.

Nothing makes a woman more beautiful than the belief she is beautiful. — Sophia Loren

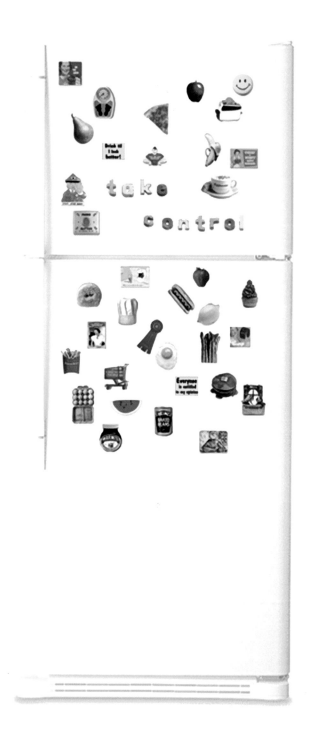

Food is an important part of a balanced diet. — Fran Lebowitz

<u>I know that sections 5 and 6 are very FACT PACKED, but don't give up. Nearly there.</u>

VARIETY IS THE SPICE OF GOOD LIFE

Back to our helpful car. We know a car does not run by petrol alone. It needs oil and water, and new brake pads when the old ones are worn out. Each element has a separate job to do towards the smooth running of the vehicle. The oil lubricates the engine, it does not cool the radiator—water does that.

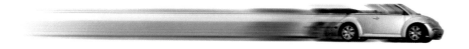

So it is with us. Our bodies have so many different running parts doing different jobs, they all need their own kind of fuel. We can find all the things we need in a varied diet. And also just like the car can't run on petrol alone, we can't run on chocolate alone for long before bits start to go wrong. It is the variety and balance from our food that will get us through an MOT.

We hear everywhere that we should be eating a 'well balanced diet', but what exactly does that mean?

There are 5 food groups:

FOOD GROUP	PURPOSE	IN WHICH FOODS
Proteins	For repairs and growth	Meat, fish, cheese, eggs, yoghurts
Carbohydrates	For energy	Bread, cereal, rice, pasta
Vitamins	For maintenance and protection	Fruit, vegetables
Calcium/minerals	For strong bones and teeth	Milk, cheese
Sugars/fats	For maintenance of organs (in small amounts) and hormones	Margarine, butter, oil, sugar

A well balanced diet would, as it implies, include a balanced amount of the first 4 groups with just a little of the 5th. Remember some foods have fewer calories for their weight so we should eat more of them and less of the more densely packed foods. Balance **doesn't** mean 200g (7oz) bread + 200g (7oz) orange + 200g (7oz) beef.

MIX AND MATCH

Foods may fit into more than one group, but for our purpose it fits into the section for which it has most of.

For example:

* A potato is mainly carbohydrate but also contains vitamins.
* Cheese is mainly protein but also contains calcium and fat.
* A banana is mainly vitamins and minerals but also contains carbohydrates.

EAT BRIGHT - EAT RIGHT

If the food you eat is mostly this colour? you are not getting enough variety in your meals! Try and get as many different colours on your plate as you can. It's good for your eyes as well as your stomach

GET THE BALANCE RIGHT

Lets look at a typical day's basic meals. As you can see from the following 3 photos, it's not the most exciting menu in the world but it is balanced.

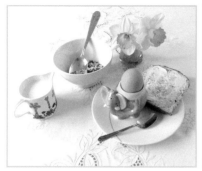 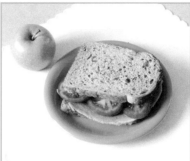 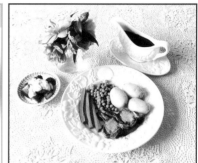

	PROTEIN	CARBOHYDRATES	VITAMINS	CALCIUM	SUGARS/FATS
BREAKFAST	egg	toast bowl of cereal		milk	sugar on cereal butter on toast
LUNCH	ham	bread	tomato apple		butter on bread
DINNER	lamb chops	potatoes	carrots peas berries	yoghurt	

We have a balance of each group throughout the day. The fats and sugars are kept to a minimum and are eaten earlier on so there is more chance of them being used up. Proteins and carbohydrates are evenly spaced through the day. We have had our recommended minimum 5 fruits and vegetables.

The most remarkable thing about my mother is that for thirty years she served the family nothing but leftovers. The original meal has never been found. — Calvin Trillin

Here's to us, my good fat friends, to bless the things we eat; for it has been full many a year, since we have seen our feet. — Anon

Now go back to 2 of your diary days and fill in the table below as we did on the previous page. See how it compares. Are you eating too many carbohydrates and fats? Are they all clustered towards the end of the day when you are less likely to exercise them off? Have you had enough fruit and vegetables?

DATE				
PROTEIN	CARBOHYDRATES	VITAMINS	CALCIUM	SUGARS/FATS

DATE				
PROTEIN	CARBOHYDRATES	VITAMINS	CALCIUM	SUGARS/FATS

Phew! That's the tough bit done.

I hope you understood sections 5 and 6. Re read them as many times as you need until you get it. There are 2 parts to achieving anything—understanding then doing. You can't do anything unless you understand it. This section is central to understanding why you are overweight and how you can get back in control of food. If you understand this bit, you can create a plan to deal with it. I know it's been a bit fact intense with not much input from you. So to check you've understood it all, have a go at this quiz. Answers on next page.

Quiz Time

1. Why do we need food?

2. What has more calories 100g (3.5oz) pizza or 100g (3.5oz) lettuce?

3. What does the body do with the food you eat?

4. Where can I find out the caloric value of a serving of baked beans?

5. What is the caloric value of a serving of baked beans?

6. If you ate 1856 kcal and used 1923 in a day, would you lose or gain weight?

7. What is the suggested minimum requirement of fruit and vegetables?

8. Which groups would the following foods go in?

| jam | courgette | lamb chop |
| spaghetti | mackerel | |

9. Why is it bad to eat a big meal late at night?

10. What happens to metabolism as you age?

11. What is a calorie?

12. Which activity uses more calories ironing or running?

13. Why is chocolate a bad option when you're feeling peckish?

14. What is the recommended daily calorie intake for a woman to maintain weight?

15. What is metabolism?

How did you do? If you got over 10 right then carry on to the next section. If you got less than 10 it might be a good idea to go over sections 5 and 6 again. Especially on the subjects you got wrong.

Answers

1. Food is the fuel our bodies use for repair, maintenance and movement.
2. Pizza has more calories.
3. The body converts food into energy.
4. The caloric value can be found on the label in the 'Nutrition Information' list.
5. A serving of baked beans (1/2 can) contains 178kcal
6. You have used 67kcal more than you have eaten, therefore, you will have lost a little.
7. 5 portions of different fruit and vegetables a day is recommended.
8. Jam (sugars) courgette (vitamins) lamb chop (protein) spaghetti (carbohydrate) mackerel (protein).
9. If you eat a large meal at night, the body does not have a chance to burn off all the calories.
10. Your metabolism slows down as you age.
11. A calories is a measurement of energy.
12. 10 minutes running uses more calories than 10 minutes ironing.
13. Chocolate has a high caloric value for its weight.
14. A woman needs approx. 2000kcal a day to maintain weight.
15. Metabolism is the rate that the body converts food into energy.

Well done is better than well said. — Benjamin Franklin

ALL THE BAD NEWS

ALL THAT GLITTERS IS NOT GOLD—PROCESSED FOOD
THE SHORT ANSWER

Processed food has lulled us into a false sense of security. It was developed to help busy working women who didn't have the time to cook from raw ingredients. But now a generation has passed, what conclusions could we draw about it?

1. We have a generation of people who don't know how to cook because they haven't had to.

2. The consumer has no control over the ingredients, their quality and their proportions put into the food by manufacturers.

3. In order to make it as appetising as possible, Processed foods tend to be very, very high in sugar, fats and salt; the 3 things we should be eating least of.
   Add that to the very high levels of overly processed ingredients like flour, where any goodness is processed out, means you've got weight gain on a stick.

notes

4. As we mentioned before, the average woman needs 2000kcal per day to maintain her weight and the average man needs 2500kcal.

MacDonald's Quarter Pounder with cheese and large fries = 928kcal (44.7g/1.6oz fat)

Tesco Deep Pan Meat Feast pizza = 1627kcal (87.9g/3.1oz fat)

KFC Bargain Bucket = 2524kcal (148.8g/5.2oz fat)

Co-op spare ribs = 553kcal (28.2g/1oz fat)

(Source: Slimming Magazine - The Complete Guide to Calories and Fat 2004)

<u>Handy Hint:</u> Get out your kitchen scales and weigh out 44.7g (1.6oz) of margarine. That's the amount of fat in your burger and chips. See if you can eat that much raw!

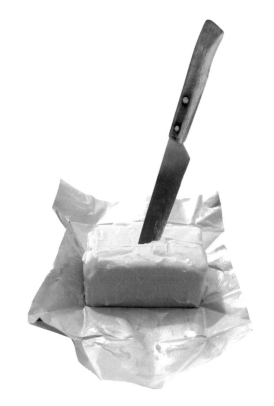

LOOK FOR YOURSELF.

5. Processed manufacturers maintain that their food is fine as part of a balanced diet. Indeed the occasional meal wouldn't do any harm. But real life isn't like that. How many days do you go through when you haven't eaten any processed food at all? Do you really cook from raw ingredients every day?

1 slice of white bread = a brisk walk for 16 mins

1 biscuit = a swim for 19 mins

I'm now at the age where I've got to prove that I'm just as good as I never was. — Rex Harrison

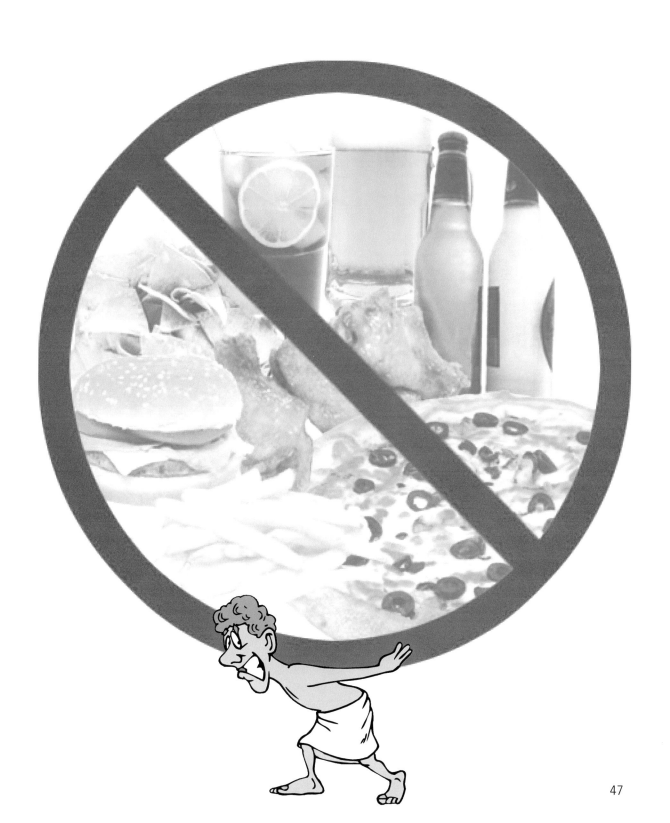

THE LONG ANSWER or MY PERSONAL RANT

I was born a post war baby and in my lifetime eating habits have changed from entirely home produced food to the processed revolution of today. We are not tied to the kitchen as our parents were. The convenience and speed that processed food gives us allows us to go out to work or do a thousand other things that aren't attached to a cooker.

However, in one generation we have lost many of the basic cooking skills that have been passed down from generation to generation. When I was a child, I remember my mother buying a whole pig. She used every single part of it. She knew how to make tongue, brawn, ox tail soup, paté, as well as bread, jam, chutney, cake etc. How many of us today can even make something as simple as short crust pastry, and then be bothered to turn it into steak and onion pie? It's so much easier to go and buy a frozen one, chuck it in the oven and greedily woof it down 45 minutes later. Unless you're really into cooking as a hobby, who's got time to make chicken Kiev or ~~lasagne~~ lasagne from scratch?

I'm no killjoy and I'm very partial to meat pie and I also don't have time to cook elaborate meals. But we must be aware of what we're eating. The advantage of processed food is the time saving convenience but the disadvantages are greater. We have no control over what goes into the food. You only have the choice to buy it or not buy it. I bet at some time you have said something like, 'there's not much chicken in this chicken hot pot'.

It's not only the main ingredients that are in the manufacturers hands. It's all the less obvious ingredients we need to be concerned with. Look for yourself on the side of a packet. Take a note of how many grams of fat, sugar and salt have been put in. They will be high. To have the very occasional processed meal is not going to do much harm, but when they become the mainstay of your diet, you will be eating too much fat, sugar and salt per day never mind overly processed ingredients such as flour. So all in all you are eating too many calories that are made up of too high a percentage of group 5 foods and other ingredients that have had a lot of their goodness ~~process~~ processed out. Doesn't sound so great put like that. Don't even get me started on crisps!

I think it's no accident that the British population was at its healthiest, ironically, during the Second World War. Foods were basic and if possible home grown to supplement short rations. I'm not saying that we should all become parsnip growers or that powdered egg was the answer to all ills, but surely we can learn a small lesson from history. <u>Processed food is not the answer to modern life.</u>

We are the luckiest generation to live. We can get fresh food from all parts of the globe all year round. We should eat more of it. And while we're at it, why not buy a simple cookbook and maybe learn some of the cooking techniques our mothers and grandmothers knew.

Finally – the big food corporations say that they are only following consumer tastes. That's you and me buying the stuff. If we didn't buy, they would stop making. If so, ask yourself truthfully, 'why do I buy processed food'? Is it the convenience? Is it because you actually can't cook? Are you addicted to the salty, fatty taste? BE HONEST. ☹

May you die in bed aged 97 shot by the jealous wife of a teenage husband. — Anon

MORE BAD NEWS

1. The first 3 days on any diet are hell. But stick with it and remember what is happening to your body. You are used to a certain amount of food. You are cutting it down dramatically and your body will not be happy about it. You will feel huge hunger pains, you may get a headache, and you may feel tired or depressed. It's just your body's way of saying, 'Oi! What's going on out there'. <u>This soon passes as you acclimatise to your new eating levels.</u>

2. You are not going to be a stick insect in one month. Think how long it has taken to get this big and this unfit. But this time you are going to lose the weight steadily and gradually and keep it off for good. Aren't you?

3. If your diet has been high in carbohydrate, fat, sugar or salt, your body will complain when they are reduced and give you mild withdrawal symptoms, but your body will re-adjust.

4. Beware! In the first week, the temptation to snack on junk or go back to old habits will be large. **Don't give in.** Don't snack on anything that contains fat or carbohydrate. Only snack enough to get rid of the hunger pains. <u>Learn to listen to your body</u> again. Feeling mildly hungry means your body is looking for fuel and will turn to the stored fat for its energy as long as you are exercising.

5. Stop eating when you've had enough. Leave the food on your plate. But when is enough? You have to learn to listen to your body again. If you feel your stomach beginning to stretch, you've gone too far. Rather than dishing up all the food straight onto the plates, may I suggest you put the food onto serving plates of some kind, then you can give yourself a little and go back for more if you need to. ☞

6. **Don't kid yourself!** It's pointless having a sneaky chocy snack or an extra glass of wine and trying to tell yourself that it doesn't matter. YES IT DOES. <u>Take responsibility for everything you put in your mouth.</u> Are you prepared to do the extra exercise to work off those extra calories? If not don't do it.

7. Same with exercise. Make a commitment to yourself that no matter what, you will put in at least 20 minutes exercise a day, 5 days a week. It's so easy to bunk off a day because you are too tired/busy/harassed/sore from yesterday's exercise. **No excuses! Do it! It's half of the diet.**

8. <u>If you fall off the wagon</u>, buy a packet of biscuits and eat them all in 30 seconds flat, do not despair. It is not the end of the world. You have not failed. You have only eaten a packet of biscuits too quickly. All you've done is put back the day you reach your ideal weight. Just get back on the diet and if you do a bit more exercise than normal you will burn off some of the extra calories anyway. More importantly, **ask yourself why** you binged. BE HONEST and try hard not to repeat the experience again, or avoid it if you can see it coming.

I learned to recognise the different stages of my hunger:

Large stomach cramps = extremely hungry, eat something

Gentle hunger pains = liveable with until the next meal

Not aware of stomach = eaten exactly the right amount

Slightly bloated feeling = eaten too much

Stretched stomach = eaten way too much, feel uncomfortable

TAKE CONTROL OF YOU

We all overeat for different reasons, amongst which are:

We're happy.

We're sad.

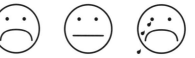

We're bored.

We're depressed.

The boyfriend just ran off with the size 8, exotic dancer who worked part time at the chippy.

The credit card took a huge battering last month because the steeplejack shop had a 50% sale on lightweight ladders.

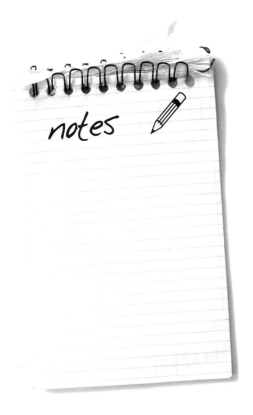

notes

They are short-term feelings that pass. If we're put under strong emotional pressure it is easy to use food as a comfort. I have no gripe with that. I know we've all done it. But get rid of/or over the problem and your eating should go back to a reasonable level.

But what happens if you find yourself in a longer-term situation that is making you miserable with no obvious way out. Perhaps it is money worries, relationship problems, personal confidence, historical issues that have never been solved or employment problems. Food can become a major crutch and then in turn, create problems of its own.

Perhaps you could use this opportunity to take an honest look at your relationship with your food.

Do you use it as a crutch for some area in your life that feels too difficult to deal with?

Perhaps you could reconsider the 'excuses' you used in Section 3 and see if something is getting in the way of you losing weight and keeping it off once and for all.

If you believe you may have personal and emotional issues its time to confront, please do not despair. There are specialists out there who will help. Please contact your doctor for initial advice. Sometimes you can't see the wood for the trees and it's hard to see where one problem starts and the next one finishes. Get any help necessary from the right people, and in the meantime, may I suggest this as a personal starting point:

You may feel you have no control over your life/job/relationships/finances/history.
But you can take control of your body and what you put in your mouth!

 # IT IS YOUR BODY. TAKE CONTROL OF IT.

Sometimes, to get control of one part of your life can help to deal with the others. I hope you find that as you lose weight and get fitter it gives you strength and confidence to find help with the other stuff.

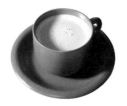

ENJOY A COFFEE BREAK

ACROSS

1. Potatoes are a _____
4. Exercise will improve your _____
6. Abbreviation for centimetre
8. Olive ____ is a type of good fat
9. Processed foods contain a lot of hidden sugar, fats and _____
10. _____ is unused energy
11. The main principle of this diet: calories ___ vs. calories out
14. A calorie is a measure of _____
15. If you consume more calories than you burn will you lose weight?
17. Exercise these regularly and you will tone up
19. Better to climb these than take the lift
20. Losing weight steadily, gradually and keeping it off is a sign of a good _____
21. The faster you run, the more calories you _____
23. By law, you will find these listed on the packaging of all food products
24. A little _____ goes a long way

DOWN

1. Consume less of these and you will lose weight
2. Standard weight meaurement system
3. Getting enough is just as important as diet and exercise
4. Abbreviation for fluid
5. Only do this when you are hungry
7. Helps moderate the rate at which the body converts food to energy
9. _____ your muscles before and after exercise
12. The bad cycle of dieting and regaining weight is called _____ dieting
13. Carrots are a type of _____
16. The science of food intake
18. To limit your intake of caffeine cut down on ____ and coffee
19. An easy and helpful to way to control how much you eat is to control _____ size
22. Drink at least 6 glasses of this a day

I intend to live forever — so far, so good. — Anon

GET DOWN AND MOVE IT

Let's reconsider the main principle of this diet:

Calories In   VS.   Calories Out
(Food)   (Activity)

If we put calories in on one side, we must use them up plus some on the other side if we want to lose weight. As we established earlier, fat is just unused energy.

We've talked at length about calories in but now we must discuss how to use up calories out through exercise. They are of equal importance here.

Just sitting around does use calories up, and so does doing our normal days activities, but nowhere near what we are putting in. That's why we're getting fat. Thus we must exercise them off and give ourselves the hidden boost of speeding up our metabolic rate. Then we'll burn off more calories without trying and we'll have more energy to cope with life.

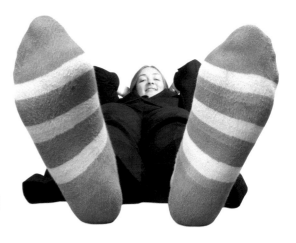

A DIET WITHOUT EXERCISE IS ONLY HALF A DIET

So, when was the last time you did any exercise?

WHICH ONE ARE YOU?

Perhaps, like me, you used to dread games lessons at school. I was tall and gangly, had little coordination, waddled rather than ran and always came last. In fact, that loathing of sport lasted till I was 41. I spent my adult life avoiding the nasty stuff. Shame really. When I did finally start to do it, I found a physical confidence that had been missing my entire life. Still, better late than never.

Or perhaps you were one of those people who were quite good at sport and managed to keep it going until your early 20's when you lost interest.

Or perhaps you were always great at sport. Always came first. Were you captain of the netball, hockey, football, long distance swimming and tiddly-winks team? You carried on doing sport until your 30's when the time demands of partners, work, house and children took their toll. You haven't done any physical activity for so long and you miss feeling fit.

However much or little you have done in the past, I am willing to bet you don't do any now. That is unless you are training to be a sumo wrestler and need the excess weight, I don't think so.

Having sex uses 8 calories a minute.

BUT HOW DO I START?

I am assuming that like me you have done little to no exercise, so we will begin at the beginning. If you are naturally sportier you can start a bit further along the line. But for anyone who hasn't done any formal exercise for over 6 months, please begin by doing 20 minutes a day, 5 days a week and gradually build it up as shown below.

```
WEEK 1 & 2  = 20 MINUTES EXERCISE PER DAY — 5 DAYS PER WEEK
WEEK 3 & 4  = 30 MINUTES EXERCISE PER DAY — 5 DAYS PER WEEK
WEEK 5 & 6  = 40 MINUTES EXERCISE PER DAY — 5 DAYS PER WEEK
WEEK 7 & 8  = 50 MINUTES EXERCISE PER DAY — 5 DAYS PER WEEK
WEEK 9 & 10 = 60 MINUTES EXERCISE PER DAY — 5 DAYS PER WEEK
WEEK 11+    = 60 MINUTES + You are ready to take up a sport!
```

That's right. In 3 months you'll be ready to go and join in a formal sport if you want to. Just decide what it is you'd like to do. Get in touch with a club and the trainers there will help you with more sport-specific exercise. For example, the type of exercise and body requirements to be good at kickboxing which needs quick explosive energy is very different from that needed to play tennis where endurance and strength are more necessary. But at least you'll be fit enough to seriously have a go. It may be a sport you loved playing years ago, or like me something you'd never done before but really fancied trying. There is a list of the most popular sports at the end of this section for you to mull over. Remember, you don't have to take up a sport. But wouldn't it be nice to be fit enough to have the choice whether to or not?

That's in the Future.

Let's deal with now.

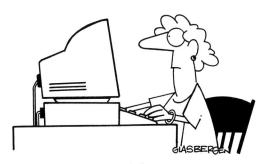

"**Welcome to the Weight Loss Forum. To lose one pound, double-click your mouse six million times.**"

WHAT KIND OF EXERCISE DO I START OFF WITH?

There are 2 types of exercise I would like you to do:

1. **Cardiovascular training**
That is anything that raises your heart rate and makes you a little breathless.

power walking

jogging

running

swimming

skipping

aerobics

cycling

rowing

jumping

climbing stairs quickly

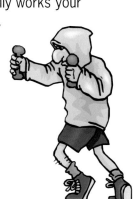

2. **Strength training**
That is anything that really works your muscles with resistance.

weightlifting

walking with weights on ankles

press ups

We will do them on <u>alternate</u> days to give your body a chance to recover and repair muscles used.

MON — Cardio
TUES — Strength
WED — Cardio
THURS — Strength
FRI — Cardio

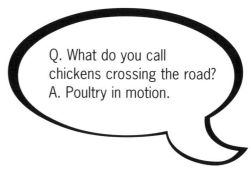

Q. What do you call chickens crossing the road?
A. Poultry in motion.

By breaking the week up I found it much easier to do and keep going. For example:

MON — 20 minutes swimming
TUES — 20 minutes weights work in room above swimming pool.
WED — 20 minutes power walking
THURS — 20 minutes ordinary walking with weight bands on ankles and wrists
FRI — 20 minutes cycling on daughter's bike

WHERE CAN I GO TO EXERCISE?

If all this is new to you, you will need to do a little research in your area to find local leisure facilities. Here's a list to get going on.

* Local libraries—ask your librarian for help. They have an encyclopedic knowledge of where to look for just about anything.
* Council/state run gyms/YMCA
* Swimming pools
* Community centres often hold classes
* Adult education centres
* Parks Department hold information of courses taking place on their properties
* Council Sport and Leisure Department.
* Private health clubs often have special offers for off-peak memberships
* Private sports clubs sometimes have general fitness training sessions.
* Internet

Exercise can lower your blood pressure, cholesterol & blood sugar.

Exercise and application produce order in affairs, health of body, cheerfulness of mind, and these make us precious to our friends. — Thomas Jefferson

To help you prepare, please make notes below of information as you gather it, of what's available, day and time it is held.

Library

Gym

Swimming Pool

Community Centre

Adult Education Centre

Parks Department

Council/State Sports and Leisure

Private Health Club

Sports Clubs

A FRIEND IN NEED...

<u>Do whatever helps to keep you motivated and doing it.</u>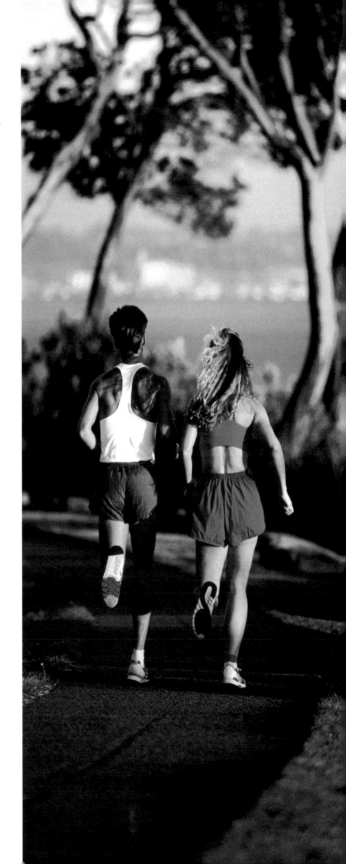

Perhaps it would suit you to find a friend and do the diet together. Exercising together can keep you both going. You can push each other to try a little harder than you would alone. You can support each other at the hopeless chocolate moments. You know the ones I mean.

Personally, I preferred to do it alone. It was precious time I had totally to myself each day. I felt I was doing something for me in my own time. After a while I joined a gym. I'd got to a point when I wanted to be amongst other people who were also trying to get fit and it helped a lot to have access to a trainer who could teach me new exercises and demand I did 10 more repetitions!

TIME IS OF THE ESSENCE

You will find it much easier to develop a daily routine and keep to it if you do your exercise at the same time of day each day. It becomes part of your normal life. If you chop and change your exercise time it becomes much easier to find an excuse not to do it that day. I found the best time for me was immediately after taking the children to school, before going to work. This may not suit you— lunchtime or after work may be more suitable.

Exuberance is beauty. — William Blake

IT'S GETTING BETTER ALL THE TIME

If you try and run a mile or weight lift 30kg (66.1lbs) straight off after having done nothing for 20 years you will:

1. Do yourself a serious damage

2. Put yourself off exercise for the rest of your life

3. Give yourself a good excuse why you can't do exercise

4. Therefore not lose any weight or get fit

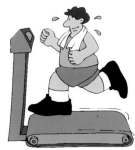

Image from clipartheaven.com

The way to do it is <u>GRADUALLY</u>. For example—running. The first time you try to run, do 30 seconds to 1 minute, followed immediately by 19 minutes walking. The next time you try, run for 2 minutes and walk for 18. The next time you run for 3 minutes and walk for 17 etc. Before you know it, you can run easily for 10 minutes. A goal you could never have done in your wildest dreams if you'd tried it on day one.

Apply this gradual process to any exercise you do. Start well inside your ability level and each time you do that activity make it a little harder or a little longer. EACH STEP MUST BE SMALL. If you cheat and jump a few steps to cut corners, it is more than likely you will pull muscles and do enough damage to stop you exercising for a few days. Then you are going backwards!

With each exercise you do, set yourself short-term goals. Such as:
At the moment I can swim 1 length without stopping—in 2 weeks I will be able to do 5 lengths.

You see? Each step can be:

Add a little more TIME

Add a little more DISTANCE

Add a little more WEIGHT

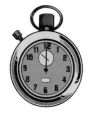
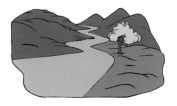
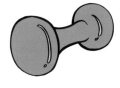

IT DOESN'T MATTER WHICH, AS LONG AS YOU HAVE GIVEN YOURSELF A REALISTIC TARGET AND EACH TIME YOU DO THE ACTIVITY, YOU MAKE IT A LITTLE HARDER THAN BEFORE

NO PAIN—NO GAIN

It's true. In order to get fit, it's going to hurt! You're using muscles that have been suffering from amnesia for a very long time. It's OK to hurt. Building muscle involves putting extra strain on it until it rips in places at a microscopic level. This is the tiredness you feel if you suddenly decide to dig the garden and can hardly move at the end of the day. Your body repairs these tears over the next 24 hours using protein you have eaten and leaving you with a slightly bigger muscle than you had before. That is why you must leave a day between exercising the same muscles.

However, you will have to learn to listen to your body again. There is a fine line between a good exercise pain and a pain that means you have gone a bit too far and done some damage. So always err on the safe side. <u>Don't injure yourself.</u> Remember, time off to recover is down time and you will have to wait until it is better before you can exercise again. Little and often is better than a lot and seldom here.

Be careful about reading health books. You may die of a misprint.
— Mark Twain

SAFE NOT SORRY

1. Always wear well fitting trainers to exercise in. They don't have to be expensive. Don't borrow other people's shoes. They mould to the feet.

2. Wear clothes you can move in easily.

3. Get goggles for swimming. These will protect your eyes from chlorine.

4. ALWAYS STRETCH YOUR MUSCLES AND WARM THEM UP BEFORE YOU EXERCISE PROPERLY TO AVOID INJURIES.

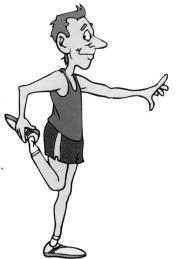

5. Don't forget to breathe deeply from the diaphragm rather than the upper chest when you exercise. To check you are doing it right—put your hand on your upper chest and breathe into it. This is shallow breathing. Now put your hand on your belly button and breathe into it. This is deep breathing.

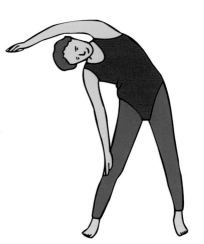

6. STRETCH YOUR MUSCLES AGAIN WHEN YOU HAVE FINISHED FORMAL EXERCISING. THIS WILL STOP YOU GETTING CRAMP.

7. When you finish exercising, don't let yourself get cold. Wrap up warm until you can shower.

8. IF YOU HAVE ANY CONCERNS AT ALL ABOUT TAKING UP EXERCISE—CONSULT YOUR DOCTOR BEFORE YOU START.

It is possible to fail in many ways... while to succeed is possible only in one way. — Aristotle

YOU EXPECT <u>ME</u> TO DO THAT!

WALK BEFORE YOU CAN RUN.

If you are more than **1 1/2 stone (9.5kg/21lbs)** overweight don't try to run till you've got down a bit. That doesn't mean you can stay a couch potato. Just start walking. This will be a huge shock to your body. Keep pushing yourself.

When you can walk easily for 20 minutes you have to push yourself to 'power walk'. That is—speed up your walking pace till you are almost jogging but not quite. It's a fast walk. Swing your hips and arms to help you get speed and momentum. It's great for your waist. To start off, see if you can power walk for 5 minutes, then reduce speed for 5 minutes to get your breath back, then speed up again then slow then fast, but never stop. You must keep moving for the full time. Eventually you will be fit enough to power walk for the full time without slowing down.

The final step is running. YOU CAN DO IT. The first time I tried, I lasted 1 minute and thought I was going to die. The next day I did 2 minutes. The next time 3 minutes and so on. I can run for an hour now. So if I did it, so can you. Could you imagine being able to run for 30 minutes? Believe me, it could be a realistic goal of yours, and achievable quicker than you think. You can also try the 'fast few minutes,' 'slow few minutes' principle as well. Whichever suits you better.

Don't forget, whichever of the above stages you start moving at, if you are feeling a bit breathless and your heart is working hard you are getting fit!

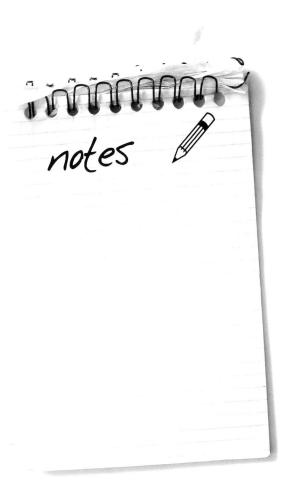

SWIM

If you can't swim—LEARN. You'll find adult classes at all pools. Don't be embarrassed or afraid. Just walk through the door, sign on the dotted line and do it. You are not the first and you won't be the last. Tell your coach of any fears you have before you get in the water. They will understand.

If you can 'leisure' swim (like you do in the holiday pool) you need to start doing some serious lengths. You may consider having a couple of lessons to help you develop your technique and to help you use your body efficiently and not put any unnecessary strain on yourself.

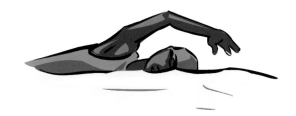

As usual, find out how many lengths you can do comfortably. Maybe it's 5. Next time you do 6 and the next 7.

AEROBICS

CLASSES

There are many aerobic classes around which you may enjoy trying. There are two basic types:

High Impact. This is when the exercise involves jumps and steps where the whole body leaves the ground. It is hard exercise and you should only attempt it if you are fit enough.

Low Impact. This is a much better option for those new to exercise. The same exercises are modified so that there is always a foot on the ground at any one time. It is still hard exercise and will tire you out if you've never tried it before. Give it a go. You may love it.

Before you join a class, ask the trainer whether it is a high or low impact class. Tell him/her about your experience so far. Good trainers always ask new members if they have any medical problems that they should know about. They should give you advice in regards to the exercises involved.

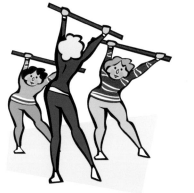 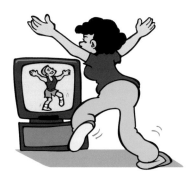

VIDEOS

There are many **aerobic videos** on the market that you may wish to try before going to a class. I have no problems with them as long as you bear the following points in mind.

1. Make sure there is enough room in front of the tele to do the programme safely.
2. Remember, the celebrity taking the class is probably already fit and if anything goes wrong they have a doctor standing just off camera. You don't. So be careful.
3. If you find a routine that suits you, you must change it after six weeks. Your body will become accustomed to the exercises and you won't be challenging it enough to get the improvements we want. So keep changing the video.
4. When you've got used to the type of exercise involved, go and join a real class. You'll get a lot more out of it.

As women age, each decade they lose 5 pounds of muscle and gain 15 pounds of fat. — Wayne Westcott, Fitness Director, YMCA, South Shore, Quiney

WEIGHTS

Weightlifting does not mean you're going to look like Schwarzenegger. It takes a HUGE amount of effort to grow muscles to that extent. I always think a great body shape is like money: damn hard to get hold of yet very easy to lose.

More realistically, what it can do is tone you up, pull in all the wobbly bits, improve your posture and if you want to slowly and gently modify your body shape, give you a way of doing it: bring your waist in, give your shoulders a stronger shape, pull your boobs up a bit!

It is a great companion activity to cardiovascular. It compliments perfectly. Each gets the bits the other one doesn't touch. However, YOU MUST DO WEIGHTS WORK UNDER SUPERVISION. Firstly, find a gym. There are many council run ones around now that are placed in leisure complexes and swimming pools. There are also many private gyms to look at. Some small and independent, others belonging to large chains. After you have joined, you will have to have a training session to show you how to use the equipment. The easiest way to start is to use the fixed machines that isolate specific muscles and work them, then when you are confident move on to free weights.

If you are new to gyms, it's hard to remember how everything works. Don't worry if you've forgotten. Go and ask the trainer on duty to jog your memory. Keep asking until you remember the basics. Don't be scared or intimidated. It's great exercise for you. Also bear in mind that all the muscly, trim people you can see in the gym weren't always like that. Everyone had to start somewhere.

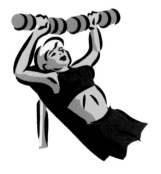 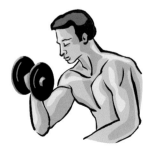

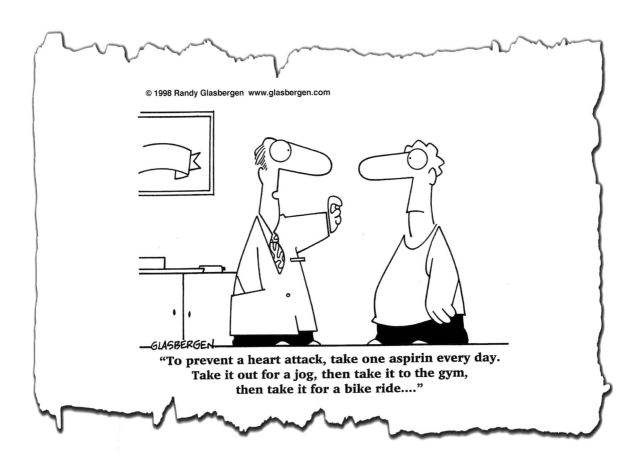

© 1998 Randy Glasbergen www.glasbergen.com

GLASBERGEN

"To prevent a heart attack, take one aspirin every day.
Take it out for a jog, then take it to the gym,
then take it for a bike ride...."

LETS GET PHYSICAL

We have taken a quick look at a few activities and how to get going with them. Of course, these may not be for you. Perhaps you will launch yourself straight into freestyle rock climbing or triathlon training. It doesn't matter what it is—as long as you do some formal exercise every day.

While we're at it, lets work on developing a more physical frame of mind. Use your body more in day-to-day life. Don't take the easy option. Make a conscious decision to move more.

TO SUM UP

1. Sticking to the exercise each day is as important as sticking to the food intake.

2. Make sure you've got the right shoes and clothes for the activity.

3. Always warm up before exercise and stretch after you've finished.

4. Whatever activity you take up—start at a level within your capabilities and make it a little harder each time you do it. Increase the level by small steps.

5. Give yourself a short-term goal, work out a daily/weekly training plan to reach your aim and stick to it. (See pages 78–81.)

6. Think active during the day. Try not to take the lazier options.

7. Do your training at the same time each day.

8. Consider doing the whole diet with a friend, you may find it easier to keep to if you do it with someone.

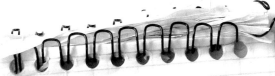

How do I move more?

- Walk up the stairs instead of using the lift.
- Walk to the shops/work/school in the morning.
- Offer to take the dog for a walk.
- Take the children to the park with a ball for half an hour and join in.
- Carry the shopping with the weight spread evenly across both hands.
- Get some rollerblades.
- Don't put off the decision to do that big physical job you've been putting off (decorating the spare room, digging the top of the garden)
- Be more selective about how much TV you watch and use some of the time doing something to improve you or your environment. It's amazing how little alterations made each day turn into big changes.

Wrinkles are hereditary. Parents get them from their children.
— Doris Day

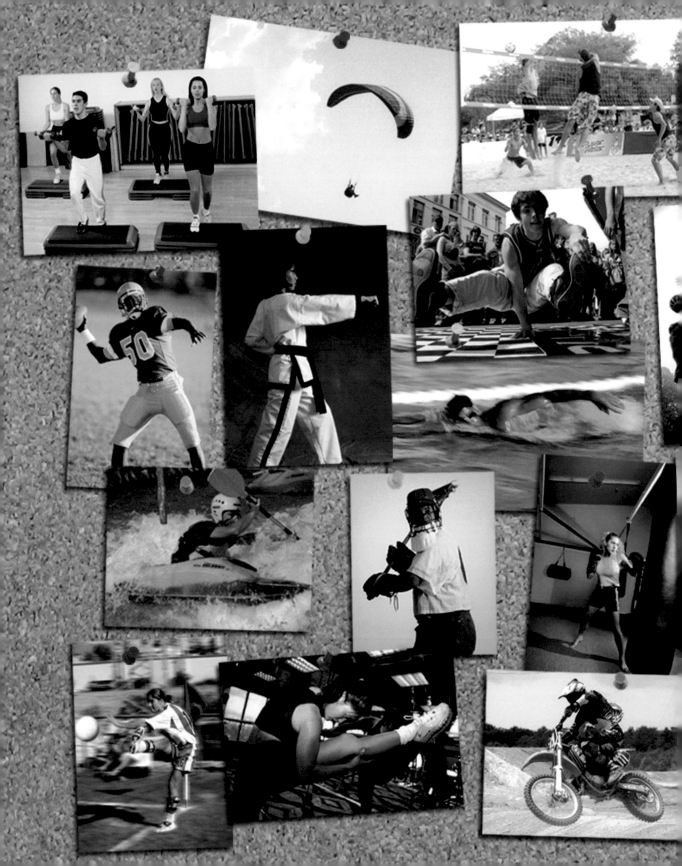

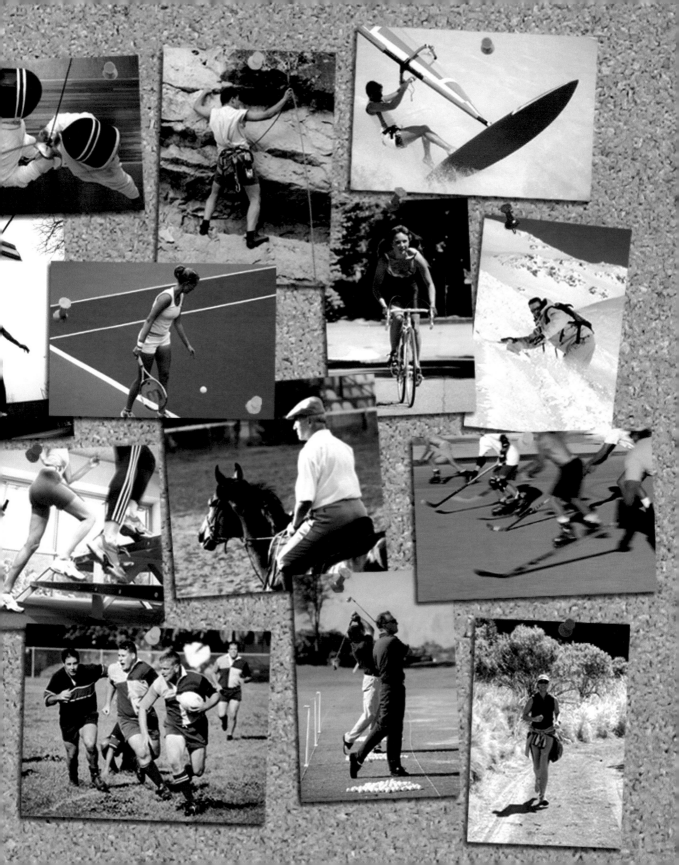

THE CHOICE IS YOURS

- Archery
- Athletics
- Aerobics
- Aqua-aerobics
- Badminton
- Baseball
- Basketball
- Bowls
- Boxing
- Canoeing
- Caving
- Cricket
- Croquet
- Cycling
- Dancing: Salsa, Ballroom, Line, Ballet, Tap, Jazz, Modern, Flamenco
- Diving
- Fencing
- Football
- Golf
- Gymnastics
- Handball
- Hiking
- Hockey (ice, street or field)
- Horseriding
- Ice Skating
- Kickboxing
- Lacrosse
- Martial Arts: Aikido, Judo, Karate, Kendo, Tae Kwon Do, Tai Chi, Tang Soo Do
- Modern Pentathlon
- Motorcycling

- Mountaineering
- Motor Racing
- Netball
- Orienteering
- Parachuting
- Pilates, Yoga
- Polo
- Rambling
- Rock Climbing
- Rollerblading
- Rollerskating
- Rowing
- Rugby
- Running (track or marathon)
- Sailing
- Shooting (clay pigeon)
- Softball
- Squash
- Sub Aqua
- Swimming
- Skateboarding
- Snowboarding
- Skiing
- Table Tennis
- Tennis
- Triathlon
- Volleyball
- Waterskiing
- Water Polo
- Windsurfing
- Wrestling
- Weightlifting

…just to name a few

You're not drunk if you can lie on the floor without holding on. — Dean Martin

REWARDING YOURSELF AND GOING OUT

In order to help keep yourself on the diet, please use this rewards system. I think you'll find it may keep you going.

DAILY REWARD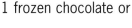

If you get through the day and have stuck to the diet (with absolutely no cheating) and have done the correct amount of exercise, at the end of the day please allow yourself either:

1 small glass of wine or   1 frozen chocolate or   1 hard boiled sweet

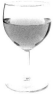   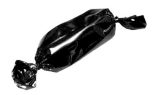

(A friend gave me this dieting tip and it worked brilliantly for me: Buy a box of single chocolates and put them in the freezer. It takes a long time to eat a single frozen chocolate!)

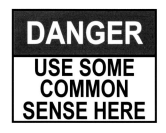

If you are a chocoholic then don't pick the frozen chocolate as your reward. If you are a bit too fond of the old vino don't pick the small glass of wine. If you think you won't be able to stop at one— then keep well away and pick something else that you would consider a small reward.

WEEKLY REWARD

If you get through the whole week and have stuck to the diet and the exercise regime without cheating, then reward yourself one night a week by having an evening meal of anything you like. It will slow your weight loss down a tiny amount but if it makes you feel good and more likely to stick to the diet for the rest of the week then, who cares.

GOING OUT

You can also use your 'one night off' to match any invitation you get to go out for a meal. You can go out and enjoy yourself without feeling guilty. Just swop the days around. However, another small caution. The reward to eat anything is more for the range of food you can pick rather than the amount. If you would normally have 3 courses at a restaurant, then keep it down to 2. Or if you are at home, you could use a dinner plate but don't attempt to eat a Mount Everest amount of food.

MONTHLY REWARD

If you get through a month without cheating, then you should give yourself a serious reward. Check to see if you've dropped a dress size yet, and if you have, go buy a little something and wear it. This will do you more good than anything and help to keep you on the diet for another month. Now you've got going—go all the way. Don't stop. If buying clothes doesn't do it for you, then get something that does. You've deserved it. What about a new hairstyle to reflect the new, energetic, younger looking you.

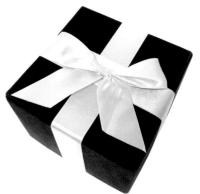

You will now have to do a revised goal list for month 2.
(Continuation packs of Exercise Plan, Short Term Goals and Weights and Measurements forms that cover 2 months per pack can be ordered from publisher. Please see order form on page 124).

You can tell a lot about a fellow's character by his way of eating jellybeans. — Ronald Reagan

SECTION 10

Early bird gets the worm, but the second mouse gets the cheese.
— Anon

IMPORTANT POINTS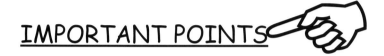

LET'S GET READY FOR THE EXERCISE

1. Make sure you have the right clothing and can move easily. Make sure you have a well fitting pair of trainers. It is better on your eyes to have goggles for swimming.

2. Have your weekly exercise plan worked out in advance. (See pages 78–81.) Make sure you know what you are going to do each day, where and at what time. Also have your short-term goals worked out.

3. Buy cheap body lotion and slap it on thickly, all over after you shower. The body will absorb as much as it needs. I found that as I lost weight my skin got a little saggy and drawn. This will help your skin shrink to fit your new shape and make you look younger and healthier for the attention you give it. I repeat, you do not need to buy expensive body lotion for this.

4. Measure and weigh yourself once a week. Do it on the same day, at the same time of day and wearing the same things. Keep a note of the changes on the chart. (page 82) Don't get fixated by weight.

5. Muscle weighs more than fat. Therefore, there will come a time when your weight loss slows down. Keep with it. It means the fat is still decreasing and muscle is increasing. You will see the changes in the tape measure not on the scales.

LET'S GET READY FOR THE FOOD

1. Go through your kitchen cupboards fridge and freezer. Separate all the high fat and processed foods. Few of us can afford to throw food away so use it up but don't replace it with more of the same. If you can afford to put it in the bin—then do it.

2. Either buy or borrow a 'low fat' cookbook. The first month on this diet uses simple basic foods, but after a while, when you get a 'feel' for the diet you might want to eat something a little more adventurous.

3. NEVER SHOP FOR FOOD WHEN YOU ARE HUNGRY. Think ahead and make sure you have all the ingredients you will need in advance. If you find that certain fresh food is more expensive than you normally buy, remember, you are cutting down on amounts. We're going for quality rather than quantity.

4. SNACKING. If you must eat between meals, stick to fruit or a few vegetables in a low fat dip or some type of protein, which will make you feel full. I found the thing that suited me best was to carry around a packet of dried mixed fruit. Only snack enough to take the hunger pain away. Snacks are not another meal. Under no circumstances eat carbohydrates. They will make you crave more.

5. Your EVENING MEAL whatever it is must be eaten on a standard 7–8" (18–20cm) tea plate. You can eat as much food as you can get on the tea plate and no more. This is very important because the size of the plate will help you to regulate the amounts.

7–8" (18–20cm)

6. Buy only skimmed or semi-skimmed milk.

7. Always go for the low fat option i.e. low fat mayonnaise, low fat dressing, low fat cottage cheese, low fat spread etc. Dump the margarine and use butter. (many margarines have hydrogenated fats in them. The worst of all!)

8. BREAD. Ban overly processed, white, sliced bread from your home. The world is full of wonderful, tasty breads. You could start with wholemeal then why not experiment with bagel, ciabatta, pitta, rye, barley and sunflower etc. They have more fibre in them. If you have a bread maker at the back of the cupboard, why not get it out and start to use it. Hey! Good Christmas pressy request.

9. Talking of banning, put the deep fat fryer in the attic. If you need to fry something, only use 1 teaspoon of oil. (olive oil is best option)

10. DRINKS. Try and reduce your intake of tea and coffee. Certainly cut in half the amount of sugar you put in hot drinks. Work towards getting rid of sugar in drinks. Try fruit teas as an option. You should also try to drink at least 6 glasses of pure water a day.

11. Don't ever miss meals. The hunger pains will make you crave the bad stuff and you might be tempted to binge. Always eat breakfast. You will not lose weight quicker by missing meals.

12. Alcohol is calorie city on a Los Angeles scale. If you must drink, keep alcohol to your daily reward.

13. Salt is now linked to high blood pressure. Cook with it if you must but keep it off the table.

14. If you are VEGETARIAN, substitute meat/fish for quorn, soya or other meat substitute of your choice.

Quit worrying about your health. It'll go away. — Robert Orben

EXERCISE PLAN

Fill in your intended exercise for each day.

EXAMPLE WEEK   *example*
MON — CARDIO   *walking round park*
TUES — STRENGTH   *weights at gym*
WED — CARDIO   *swim*
THURS — STRENGTH   *walk with ankle and wrist weights*
FRI — CARDIO   *bicycle to Neston Village and back*

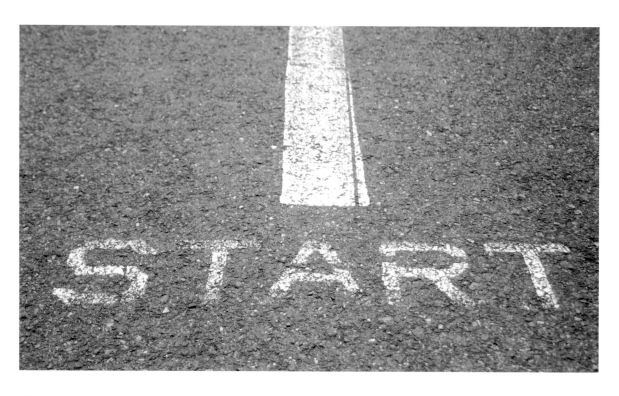

WEEK 1

MON — CARDIO

TUES — STRENGTH

WED — CARDIO

THURS — STRENGTH

FRI — CARDIO

WEEK 2

MON — CARDIO

TUES — STRENGTH

WED — CARDIO

THURS — STRENGTH

FRI — CARDIO

WEEK 3

MON — CARDIO

TUES — STRENGTH

WED — CARDIO

THURS — STRENGTH

FRI — CARDIO

WEEK 4

MON — CARDIO

TUES — STRENGTH

WED — CARDIO

THURS — STRENGTH

FRI — CARDIO

Happiness is nothing more than good health and a bad memory.
— Albert Schweitzer

SHORT TERM GOALS

SOME EXAMPLES

ACTIVITY	DATE	CAN DO NOW	GOAL	ACHIEVED
Swimming	14/3/06	3 lengths	6 lengths	21/3/06
Running	15/3/06	0	5 mins	30/3/06
Star jumps	16/3/06	2	10	
Swimming	30/3/06	6 lengths	15 lengths	

SHORT TERM GOALS continued

ACTIVITY	DATE	CAN DO NOW	GOAL	ACHIEVED

I never eat on an empty stomach. — Tallulah Bankhead

WEIGHTS AND MEASUREMENTS

STARTING WEIGHT					
START DATE			END DATE		
END OF...	WEEK 1	WEEK 2	WEEK 3	WEEK 4	**TOTAL LOSS**
WEIGHT					
NECK					
CHEST					
WAIST					
HIPS					
THIGHS					
KNEES					

Continuation packs of Exercise Plan, Short Term Goals and Weights and Measurements forms that cover 2 months per pack can be ordered from publisher. Please see order form on page 124.

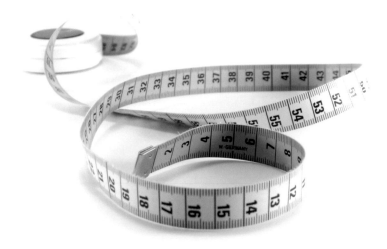

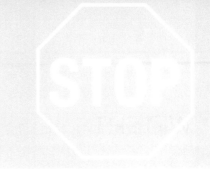

YOU <u>WILL BE</u> WHAT YOU EAT

The diet you are about to start is unashamedly straightforward and simple and I make no apologies for it. The reason being that it directly addresses many of the lifestyle issues discussed earlier that help cause obesity:

PROBLEM	SOLUTION
1. A reliance on processed food	1. This diet uses simple, basic foods with as little processed food as possible
2. A generation who have lost the skills to cook	2. The daily programme gives the dieter a chance to learn how to cook simple yet hearty, healthy meals
3. People do not have time to prepare elaborate meals	3. The simplicity of the menus takes no longer to cook than comparable processed meals

WARNING
Do not start this diet without working through sections 1–10. Do not let this be another yo-yo diet on your list. Once and for all find out how YOU can lose weight and keep it off.

WARNING
If your BMI is over 30 (see page 2), please see your doctor, as you may initially need more calories per day than suggested here. This should not stop you following the diet/exercise regime—please consult your doctor or a qualified practitioner for further advice.

What if I don't like what you've chosen because I don't like specific foods or I'm allergic to certain things or any other reason?

Simple. Then change it to something you do like—but stick to the principle of the diet. i.e. I picked lamb and salad. You don't like lamb—so eat steak or chicken in its place.

What if after the first week I haven't lost any weight?

If you are not losing any weight, just apply the principle of the diet—you need to either eat a bit less than suggested or do more exercise than you are doing or a little of both. We are all different and you need to find where your own personal balance of calories in and calories out is.

What do I do after the first month is over?

I hope you will gather as you follow this programme through, that there is no specific end to this diet. It is a change of life for you. It is the start of the healthier, fitter you. Please keep up the exercise 5 times a week until you reach your ideal weight. Only then can you move to a maintenance programme of 3 times a week for a minimum of an hour each time. The diet of healthy balanced low fat foods with little processed food should be seen as your normal eating regime. Keep an eye on the amounts you eat. REMEMBER THAT PILES OF GOOD HEALTHY FOOD WILL STILL MAKE YOU FAT IF YOU DON'T BURN IT OFF. You may find it helpful for the first 3 to 4 months to redo your exercise regime on paper each month with short-term goals and work out in advance what you will eat for at least a week ahead. This will help you carry on doing the exercise and will help stop you doing any binge eating.

What if I start to put weight on again slowly in the future?

Then stop it. You now know why your weight is creeping up and you know how to stop it. Be in control of it for the long term.

You should have your exercise regime all worked out and ready to go and here to complement it is the diet. Please fill in details each day as you do it. Remember all the rules, but above all… YOU are in control of what you put in your mouth.

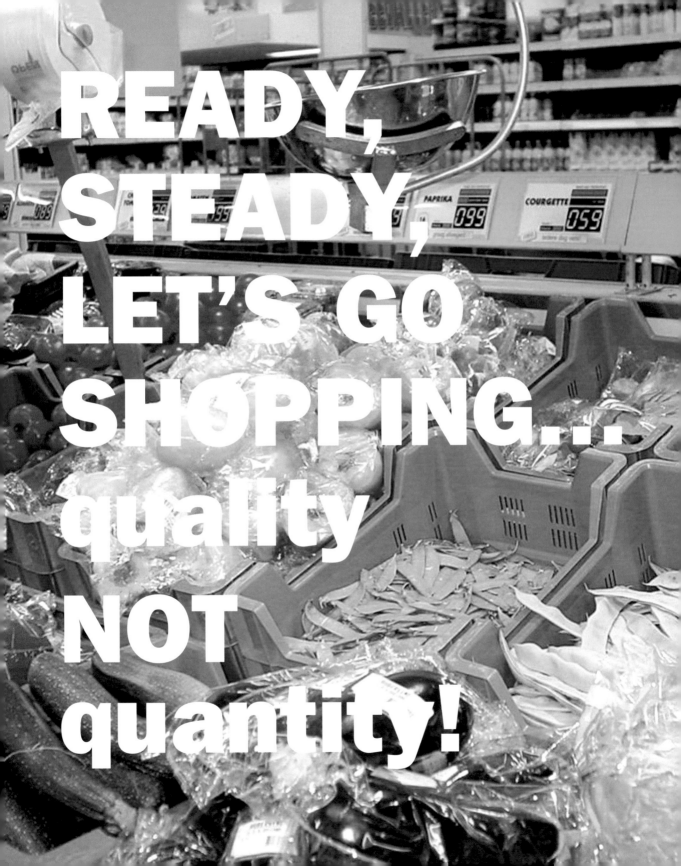

WEEK 1 SHOPPING LIST

Here is a list of ingredients you will need for the week. I have left out amounts as I don't know how many people you are cooking for. Don't forget to substitute the things you don't like i.e. chicken for lamb etc. Other things like 'sugar' you may already have.

- [ ] Box of high fibre cereal i.e. Shredded Wheat, All Bran, Weetabix (no high sugar)
- [ ] Pack of spaghetti
- [ ] Pack of other type of dried pasta
- [ ] Rice (brown is better for you than white)
- [ ] Crispbreads/cheese biscuits
- [ ] Interesting bread (not white processed)—buy fresh as needed

- [ ] Fruit: bananas, apples, oranges, baking apples + as many other fresh fruits as you like
- [ ] Vegetables: 4 different types of vegetable, baking potatoes, mushrooms, cooking onions
- [ ] Salad: lettuce, cucumber, tomatoes, celery, peppers
- [ ] Tomato based pasta sauce
- [ ] Pack dried fruit for snacks
- [ ] A few currants or sultanas
- [ ] Fruit juice

- [ ] White fish
- [ ] Ham
- [ ] Scotch egg
- [ ] Tin tuna in brine
- [ ] Chicken
- [ ] Sunday roast of your choice
- [ ] Pork (optional)
- [ ] Bacon (optional)
- [ ] Pate
- [ ] Tin baked beans

- [ ] Parsley sauce mix or make your own
- [ ] Summer pudding
- [ ] Meringue nests
- [ ] Jelly
- [ ] Fruit juice
- [ ] Jam or marmalade
- [ ] Gravy mix
- [ ] Low fat mayonnaise/low fat salad dressing

- [ ] Skimmed or semi-skimmed milk
- [ ] Low fat yoghurt desserts
- [ ] Cottage cheese/cheddar cheese
- [ ] Low fat dip
- [ ] Eggs
- [ ] Oxo or vegetable cubes + vegetable soup mix

DAY 1 Monday

 What I ate & drank, including alternatives

BREAKFAST
1 bowl cereal
Skimmed milk
1 tsp sugar

SNACK (OPTIONAL)
Crispbread
Ham

LUNCH
In a cereal bowl
Homemade pasta salad
Cook pasta and cool. Add tuna, tomato, sweetcorn and any other vegetables preferred. Before eating, mix with a little low fat salad dressing.

SNACK (OPTIONAL)
Apple

DINNER
On tea plate
Chicken
2 vegetables (no potatoes)
A little gravy
Low fat yoghurt dessert

END OF DAY REWARD ☆
Small glass of wine or
1 frozen chocolate or
1 boiled sweet

WHAT DID YOU DRINK TODAY AND HOW MUCH? DID YOU EXERCISE?		
Tea and/or coffee?	Y / N	Amount:
Juice/sweetened/fizzy drinks?	Y / N	Amount:
Water?	Y / N	Amount:
Exercise?	Y / N	I did:

DAY 2 Tuesday

BREAKFAST
1 piece toast
Jam—no butter
Fruit juice

SNACK (OPTIONAL)
Banana

LUNCH
1 bowl of chunky vegetable soup
1 chunky piece of bread

SNACK (OPTIONAL)
Scotch egg

DINNER
On tea plate
Grilled white fish
2 vegetables—no potatoes
A little parsley sauce
Baked apple stuffed with
Currants and sultanas

END OF DAY REWARD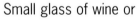
Small glass of wine or
1 frozen chocolate or
1 boiled sweet

 What I ate & drank, including alternatives

WHAT DID YOU DRINK TODAY AND HOW MUCH? DID YOU EXERCISE?		
Tea and/or coffee?	Y / N	Amount:
Juice/sweetened/fizzy drinks?	Y / N	Amount:
Water?	Y / N	Amount:
Exercise?	Y / N	I did:

DAY 3 Wednesday

 What I ate & drank, including alternatives

BREAKFAST
Bowl of mixed fresh fruit (4 kinds) covered with
Fruit yoghurt

SNACK (OPTIONAL)
Crispbread
Cottage cheese

LUNCH
Sticks of carrot, cucumber, peppers, sugar snap
peas etc.—as much as you want
Low fat dip

SNACK (OPTIONAL)
Apple

DINNER
On tea plate
Baked potato with baked beans
A little grated cheese on top—grilled
Side salad
Summer pudding

END OF DAY REWARD ⭐
Small glass of wine or
1 frozen chocolate or
1 boiled sweet

WHAT DID YOU DRINK TODAY AND HOW MUCH? DID YOU EXERCISE?		
Tea and/or coffee?	Y / N	Amount:
Juice/sweetened/fizzy drinks?	Y / N	Amount:
Water?	Y / N	Amount:
Exercise?	Y / N	I did:

DAY 4 Thursday

BREAKFAST
Boiled egg
1 piece bread
Fruit juice

SNACK (OPTIONAL)
Banana

LUNCH
Bread roll
Pate

SNACK (OPTIONAL)
4 pieces dried fruit

DINNER
On tea plate
Spaghetti
Tomato pasta sauce
Side salad
Meringue nest with
Fruit and
Yoghurt

END OF DAY REWARD
Small glass of wine or
1 frozen chocolate or
1 boiled sweet

What I ate & drank, including alternatives

WHAT DID YOU DRINK TODAY AND HOW MUCH? DID YOU EXERCISE?		
Tea and/or coffee?	Y / N	Amount:
Juice/sweetened/fizzy drinks?	Y / N	Amount:
Water?	Y / N	Amount:
Exercise?	Y / N	I did:

DAY 5 Friday

 What I ate & drank, including alternatives

BREAKFAST
1 bowl cereal
Skimmed milk
1 tsp sugar

SNACK (OPTIONAL)
Banana

LUNCH
Ham salad sandwich with
Low fat mayonnaise—no butter

SNACK (OPTIONAL)
Apple

DINNER
On tea plate
Pork/chicken stroganoff (serves 2)
*Fry 175g (6oz) meat and chopped onion in 1 tsp oil
until golden brown. Stir in 12g (1/2oz) plain flour.
Pour in 220ml (1/2 pint) stock. Stir in 1 tbsp tomato
puree. Add 65g (2 1/2oz) mushrooms 1/2 green
pepper and nutmeg to taste. Season. Bring to boil.
Reduce heat and simmer for 20 mins. Take off heat
and stir in 2 tbsp yoghurt. Serve on a bed of rice.
Sprinkle with chopped parsley.*

END OF DAY REWARD
Small glass of wine or
1 frozen chocolate or
1 boiled sweet

WHAT DID YOU DRINK TODAY AND HOW MUCH? DID YOU EXERCISE?		
Tea and/or coffee?	Y / N	Amount:
Juice/sweetened/fizzy drinks?	Y / N	Amount:
Water?	Y / N	Amount:
Exercise?	Y / N	I did:

DAY 6 Saturday

BREAKFAST
1 piece cheese or jam/honey on
1 piece toast
Fruit juice

 What I ate & drank, including alternatives

SNACK (OPTIONAL)
Banana

LUNCH
Homemade parsnip and apple soup
*Roughly chop onion. Fry in 1 tsp oil. Add 500ml
(1 pint) stock. Add 2 parsnips and 1 cooking
apple. Cook until parsnips are soft. Put in blender
and blend until smooth. Season.*

SNACK (OPTIONAL)
Crispbread with
Cottage cheese

DINNER ☆ ☆
Weekly reward
Y O U   C H O O S E !

END OF DAY REWARD ☆
Small glass of wine or
1 frozen chocolate or
1 boiled sweet

WHAT DID YOU DRINK TODAY AND HOW MUCH? DID YOU EXERCISE?		
Tea and/or coffee?	Y / N	Amount:
Juice/sweetened/fizzy drinks?	Y / N	Amount:
Water?	Y / N	Amount:
Exercise?	Y / N	I did:

DAY 7 Sunday

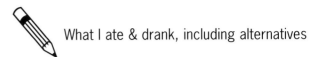
What I ate & drank, including alternatives

BREAKFAST
1 bagel or bread roll filled with
Bacon or cheese

SNACK (OPTIONAL)
Banana

LUNCH
On tea plate—Sunday roast
Meat
3 vegetables +
1 small potato
Gravy
Jelly with
Real fresh fruit inside

NO SNACK

DINNER
4 cheese biscuits with
A little cheese or pate
Grapes

END OF DAY REWARD
Small glass of wine or
1 frozen chocolate or
1 boiled sweet

**DON'T FORGET TO FILL IN YOUR WEEKLY
WEIGHTS AND MEASURES CHART.**

WHAT DID YOU DRINK TODAY AND HOW MUCH? DID YOU EXERCISE?		
Tea and/or coffee?	Y / N	Amount:
Juice/sweetened/fizzy drinks?	Y / N	Amount:
Water?	Y / N	Amount:
Exercise?	Y / N	I did:

WEEK 2 SHOPPING LIST

- [ ] Box of high fibre cereal i.e. Shredded Wheat, All Bran, Cornflakes (no high sugar or chocolate flavoured)
- [ ] Danish or breakfast cake—buy fresh as needed
- [ ] Small pack crumpets
- [ ] Crispbread
- [ ] Interesting bread (not white processed)
- [ ] Rice
- [ ] Dried pasta

- [ ] Fruit: bananas, apples, baking apple, oranges + other seasonal fresh fruits as you like
- [ ] Pack dried fruit for snacks
- [ ] Vegetables: 4 different types of vegetable + potatoes, garlic, tin of sweetcorn, onions
- [ ] Salad: lettuce, cucumber, tomatoes, celery, peppers
- [ ] Fruit juice

- [ ] Fish of your choice for grilling
- [ ] Prawns
- [ ] Lamb chops
- [ ] Quiche
- [ ] Sunday roast of your choice
- [ ] Taramasalata
- [ ] Tin baked beans
- [ ] Ham/salami

- [ ] Skimmed or semi-skimmed milk
- [ ] Mozzarella
- [ ] Low fat yoghurt desserts
- [ ] Cottage cheese
- [ ] Fromage frais
- [ ] Eggs
- [ ] Tin low fat rice pudding

- [ ] Packet low fat vegetable soup mix
- [ ] Tin of soup any variety
- [ ] Parsley sauce mix
- [ ] Meringue nests
- [ ] Jam or marmalade
- [ ] Runny honey
- [ ] Low fat mayonnaise
- [ ] Low fat salad dressing
- [ ] Gravy mix
- [ ] Olive oil
- [ ] Small ice-cream
- [ ] Jelly

DAY 8 Monday

BREAKFAST
1 Danish or
Breakfast cake

NO SNACK

LUNCH
Bowl soup—any variety (preferably homemade)
1 chunk bread

SNACK (OPTIONAL)
Crispbread with
Cottage cheese

DINNER
On tea plate
Mozzarella salad
*Cut slices of mozzarella, slices of beef tomato
and slices of ham or salami. Interweave on plate.
Sprinkle with fresh basil. Drizzle olive oil over.
Eat with…*
1 chunk bread
Low fat yoghurt dessert

END OF DAY REWARD
Small glass of wine or
1 frozen chocolate or
1 boiled sweet

 What I ate & drank, including alternatives

WHAT DID YOU DRINK TODAY AND HOW MUCH? DID YOU EXERCISE?		
Tea and/or coffee?	Y / N	Amount:
Juice/sweetened/fizzy drinks?	Y / N	Amount:
Water?	Y / N	Amount:
Exercise?	Y / N	I did:

DAY 9 Tuesday

 What I ate & drank, including alternatives

BREAKFAST
1 bowl cereal
Skimmed milk
1 tsp sugar
1 boiled egg +
1 piece of bread

NO SNACK

LUNCH
Sticks of various fresh fruit—dip into
Yoghurt with honey on it

SNACK (OPTIONAL)
Crispbread with
Cottage cheese or ham

DINNER
On tea plate
2 lamb chops
2 vegetables—no potatoes
Gravy
Meringue nest with
1 chopped fruit and
Fromage frais

END OF DAY REWARD
Small glass of wine or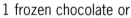
1 frozen chocolate or
1 boiled sweet

WHAT DID YOU DRINK TODAY AND HOW MUCH? DID YOU EXERCISE?		
Tea and/or coffee?	Y / N	Amount:
Juice/sweetened/fizzy drinks?	Y / N	Amount:
Water?	Y / N	Amount:
Exercise?	Y / N	I did:

DAY 10 Wednesday

BREAKFAST
Bowl of mixed fresh fruit (4 kinds) covered with
Fruit yoghurt

 What I ate & drank, including alternatives

NO SNACK

LUNCH
Salad sandwich
As much mixed salad as you can get between
2 pieces of bread. No butter—use
Mayonnaise

SNACK (OPTIONAL)
Crispbread with
Cottage cheese or ham

DINNER
On tea plate
Stuffed tomatoes
Side salad
Remove insides from beef tomatoes. Cook rice.
Mix into rice fried onion, garlic, sweetcorn,
fried bacon bits, peas—in fact anything you want
to add. Season. Stuff tomatoes with rice mixture
and bake in oven until tomatoes are softened.
Yoghurt dessert

END OF DAY REWARD
Small glass of wine or
1 frozen chocolate or
1 boiled sweet

WHAT DID YOU DRINK TODAY AND HOW MUCH? DID YOU EXERCISE?		
Tea and/or coffee?	Y / N	Amount:
Juice/sweetened/fizzy drinks?	Y / N	Amount:
Water?	Y / N	Amount:
Exercise?	Y / N	I did:

DAY 11 Thursday

BREAKFAST
2 scrambled eggs
1 piece toast—no butter

NO SNACK

LUNCH
Bowl chicken/prawn salad with
Salad dressing

SNACK (OPTIONAL)
4 pieces dried fruit

DINNER
On tea plate
Grilled fish
2 vegetables
Parsley sauce
Small bowl of rice pudding

END OF DAY REWARD
Small glass of wine or
1 frozen chocolate or
1 boiled sweet

What I ate & drank, including alternatives

WHAT DID YOU DRINK TODAY AND HOW MUCH? DID YOU EXERCISE?		
Tea and/or coffee?	Y / N	Amount:
Juice/sweetened/fizzy drinks?	Y / N	Amount:
Water?	Y / N	Amount:
Exercise?	Y / N	I did:

DAY 12 Friday

BREAKFAST
1 piece toast
Jam/marmalade
Fruit juice

NO SNACK

LUNCH
1 bowl of pasta, prawn and apple salad

SNACK (OPTIONAL)
Banana

DINNER
On tea plate
Quiche
Baked beans
Baked apple with
Small scoop of ice-cream

END OF DAY REWARD
Small glass of wine or
1 frozen chocolate or
1 boiled sweet

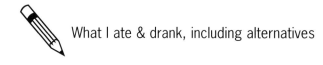
What I ate & drank, including alternatives

WHAT DID YOU DRINK TODAY AND HOW MUCH? DID YOU EXERCISE?		
Tea and/or coffee?	Y / N	Amount:
Juice/sweetened/fizzy drinks?	Y / N	Amount:
Water?	Y / N	Amount:
Exercise?	Y / N	I did:

DAY 13 Saturday

What I ate & drank, including alternatives

BREAKFAST
2 crumpets
Jam

NO SNACK

LUNCH
Bowl of garlic mash
Boil and mash potatoes. Add fried onion, garlic, parsley and fromage frais. Season. Top with
Poached egg

NO SNACK

DINNER
Weekly reward
Y O U   C H O O S E !

END OF DAY REWARD
Small glass of wine or
1 frozen chocolate or
1 boiled sweet

WHAT DID YOU DRINK TODAY AND HOW MUCH? DID YOU EXERCISE?			
Tea and/or coffee?	Y / N	Amount:	
Juice/sweetened/fizzy drinks?	Y / N	Amount:	
Water?	Y / N	Amount:	
Exercise?	Y / N	I did:	

DAY 14 Sunday

BREAKFAST
1 bagel or bread roll filled with
Bacon or cheese

NO SNACK

LUNCH
On tea plate—Sunday roast
Meat
3 vegetables +
1 small potato
Gravy
Jelly with
Real fresh fruit inside

NO SNACK

DINNER
1 pitta bread or roll with
Taramasalata and tomato

END OF DAY REWARD
Small glass of wine or
1 frozen chocolate or
1 boiled sweet

**DON'T FORGET TO FILL IN YOUR WEEKLY
WEIGHTS AND MEASURES CHART.**

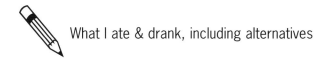
What I ate & drank, including alternatives

WHAT DID YOU DRINK TODAY AND HOW MUCH? DID YOU EXERCISE?		
Tea and/or coffee?	Y / N	Amount:
Juice/sweetened/fizzy drinks?	Y / N	Amount:
Water?	Y / N	Amount:
Exercise?	Y / N	I did:

WEEK 3 SHOPPING LIST

- [ ] Porridge oats
- [ ] Box of high fibre cereal i.e. Shredded Wheat, All Bran, Cornflakes
  (no high sugar or chocolate flavoured)
- [ ] Danish or breakfast cake—buy as needed
- [ ] Pitta bread
- [ ] Interesting bread (not white processed)
- [ ] Rice

- [ ] Fruit: bananas, apples, oranges, + other fresh fruits as you like
- [ ] Vegetables: 4 different types of vegetable + potatoes, baking potato
- [ ] Salad: lettuce, cucumber, tomatoes, celery, peppers, cress
- [ ] Fruit juice

- [ ] Skimmed or semi-skimmed milk
- [ ] Low fat yoghurt desserts
- [ ] Low fat dips
- [ ] Cottage cheese
- [ ] Fromage Frais
- [ ] Greek style yoghurt
- [ ] Eggs
- [ ] Meringue nests
- [ ] Tin low fat rice pudding
- [ ] Oven chips—small
- [ ] Chutney
- [ ] Jam or marmalade
- [ ] Honey
- [ ] Low fat mayonnaise
- [ ] Low fat salad dressing
- [ ] Gravy mix
- [ ] Ice-cream—small

- [ ] Salmon steak
- [ ] Steak
- [ ] Chicken
- [ ] Sunday roast of your choice
- [ ] Cooked ham
- [ ] Tin baked beans
- [ ] Slice gala pie or pork pie
- [ ] Sausages (good quality)
- [ ] Cheddar cheese

DAY 15 Monday

BREAKFAST
1 boiled egg
1 piece of toast

NO SNACK

LUNCH
Mixed vegetable fingers with
Low fat dips
banana

NO SNACK

DINNER
On tea plate
Chicken
2 vegetables
Gravy
Low fat yoghurt dessert

END OF DAY REWARD
Small glass of wine or
1 frozen chocolate or
1 boiled sweet

What I ate & drank, including alternatives

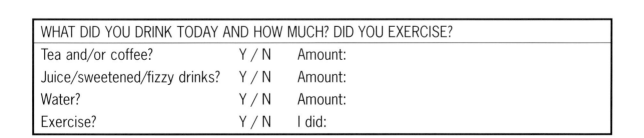

WHAT DID YOU DRINK TODAY AND HOW MUCH? DID YOU EXERCISE?		
Tea and/or coffee?	Y / N	Amount:
Juice/sweetened/fizzy drinks?	Y / N	Amount:
Water?	Y / N	Amount:
Exercise?	Y / N	I did:

DAY 16 Tuesday

BREAKFAST
1 bowl cereal
Skimmed milk
1 tsp sugar

NO SNACK

LUNCH
Large fresh fruit salad with
Greek style yoghurt

NO SNACK

DINNER
On tea plate
Baked potato
Baked beans
Topped with grilled grated cheese
Meringue nest with
1 chopped fruit and
Fromage frais

END OF DAY REWARD
Small glass of wine or
1 frozen chocolate or
1 boiled sweet

 What I ate & drank, including alternatives

WHAT DID YOU DRINK TODAY AND HOW MUCH? DID YOU EXERCISE?		
Tea and/or coffee?	Y / N	Amount:
Juice/sweetened/fizzy drinks?	Y / N	Amount:
Water?	Y / N	Amount:
Exercise?	Y / N	I did:

DAY 17 Wednesday

BREAKFAST
1 danish pastry or
Breakfast cake

NO SNACK

LUNCH
Egg mayonnaise with cress in
1 roll

NO SNACK

DINNER
On tea plate
Steak and oven chips with
Side salad
Yoghurt dessert

END OF DAY REWARD ☆
Small glass of wine or
1 frozen chocolate or
1 boiled sweet

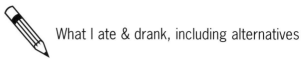 What I ate & drank, including alternatives

WHAT DID YOU DRINK TODAY AND HOW MUCH? DID YOU EXERCISE?		
Tea and/or coffee?	Y / N	Amount:
Juice/sweetened/fizzy drinks?	Y / N	Amount:
Water?	Y / N	Amount:
Exercise?	Y / N	I did:

DAY 18 Thursday

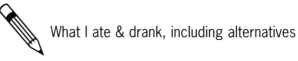 What I ate & drank, including alternatives

BREAKFAST
Bowl hot porridge
Skimmed milk
1 tsp sugar

NO SNACK

LUNCH
Ham salad

NO SNACK

DINNER
On tea plate
2 sausages
Mash
1 green vegetable
Small bowl of rice pudding

END OF DAY REWARD ☆
Small glass of wine or
1 frozen chocolate or
1 boiled sweet

WHAT DID YOU DRINK TODAY AND HOW MUCH? DID YOU EXERCISE?		
Tea and/or coffee?	Y / N	Amount:
Juice/sweetened/fizzy drinks?	Y / N	Amount:
Water?	Y / N	Amount:
Exercise?	Y / N	I did:

DAY 19 Friday

BREAKFAST
1 piece toast
Jam/marmalade
Fruit juice

NO SNACK

LUNCH
Pitta bread stuffed with
Chicken, tomato and
Mayonnaise

NO SNACK

DINNER
On tea plate
Steamed or grilled salmon
2 vegetables
2 scoops of ice-cream

END OF DAY REWARD
Small glass of wine or
1 frozen chocolate or
1 boiled sweet

What I ate & drank, including alternatives

WHAT DID YOU DRINK TODAY AND HOW MUCH? DID YOU EXERCISE?		
Tea and/or coffee?	Y / N	Amount:
Juice/sweetened/fizzy drinks?	Y / N	Amount:
Water?	Y / N	Amount:
Exercise?	Y / N	I did:

DAY 20 Saturday

BREAKFAST
Cereal
Skimmed milk
1 tsp sugar

NO SNACK

LUNCH
Homemade soup of your choice
1 chunk bread

NO SNACK

DINNER ☆☆
Weekly reward
Y O U   C H O O S E !

END OF DAY REWARD ☆
Small glass of wine or
1 frozen chocolate or
1 boiled sweet

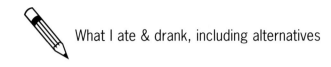 What I ate & drank, including alternatives

WHAT DID YOU DRINK TODAY AND HOW MUCH? DID YOU EXERCISE?		
Tea and/or coffee?	Y / N	Amount:
Juice/sweetened/fizzy drinks?	Y / N	Amount:
Water?	Y / N	Amount:
Exercise?	Y / N	I did:

DAY 21 Sunday

BREAKFAST
1 bagel or bread roll
Filled with jam or bacon or cheese

NO SNACK

LUNCH
On tea plate—Sunday roast
Meat
3 vegetables +
1 small potato
Gravy
Dessert of your choice

NO SNACK

DINNER
Slice gala/pork pie
Tomatoes
Chutney

END OF DAY REWARD
Small glass of wine or
1 frozen chocolate or
1 boiled sweet

**DON'T FORGET TO FILL IN YOUR WEEKLY
WEIGHTS AND MEASURES CHART.**

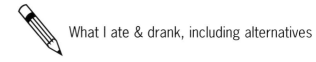

What I ate & drank, including alternatives

WHAT DID YOU DRINK TODAY AND HOW MUCH? DID YOU EXERCISE?		
Tea and/or coffee?	Y / N	Amount:
Juice/sweetened/fizzy drinks?	Y / N	Amount:
Water?	Y / N	Amount:
Exercise?	Y / N	I did:

WEEK 4 SHOPPING LIST

- [ ] Box of high fibre cereal i.e. Shredded Wheat, All Bran, Cornflakes
  (no high sugar or chocolate flavoured)
- [ ] Danish or breakfast cake
- [ ] Crispbread
- [ ] Interesting bread (not white processed)
- [ ] Spaghetti

- [ ] Fruit: bananas, apples, oranges + other fresh fruits as you like
- [ ] Vegetables: 4 different types of vegetables + potatoes, baking potato
- [ ] Salad: lettuce, cucumber, tomatoes, celery, peppers
- [ ] Fruit juice

- [ ] Lamb chops
- [ ] Mince for bolognese
- [ ] Sunday roast of your choice
- [ ] Tin tuna in brine

- [ ] Skimmed or semi-skimmed milk
- [ ] Low fat yoghurt desserts
- [ ] Eggs
- [ ] Cheese
- [ ] Meringue nests
- [ ] Tin/packet soup
- [ ] Gravy mix
- [ ] Low fat mayonnaise
- [ ] Low fat salad dressing

DAY 22 Monday

BREAKFAST
Cereal
Skimmed milk
1 tsp sugar
Glass fruit juice

NO SNACK

LUNCH
Cheese salad sandwich

NO SNACK

DINNER
On tea plate
Spaghetti bolognese
Meringue nests with
Fruit and
Yoghurt

END OF DAY REWARD ☆
Small glass of wine or
1 frozen chocolate or
1 boiled sweet

 What I ate & drank, including alternatives

WHAT DID YOU DRINK TODAY AND HOW MUCH? DID YOU EXERCISE?		
Tea and/or coffee?	Y / N	Amount:
Juice/sweetened/fizzy drinks?	Y / N	Amount:
Water?	Y / N	Amount:
Exercise?	Y / N	I did:

DAY 23 Tuesday

 What I ate & drank, including alternatives

BREAKFAST
2 eggs boiled or scrambled
1 piece bread

NO SNACK

LUNCH
Bowl soup
1 chunk bread

NO SNACK

DINNER
On tea plate
Baked potato
Tuna mayonnaise
Side salad
Yoghurt dessert

END OF DAY REWARD
Small glass of wine or
1 frozen chocolate or
1 boiled sweet

WHAT DID YOU DRINK TODAY AND HOW MUCH? DID YOU EXERCISE?		
Tea and/or coffee?	Y / N	Amount:
Juice/sweetened/fizzy drinks?	Y / N	Amount:
Water?	Y / N	Amount:
Exercise?	Y / N	I did:

DAY 24 Wednesday

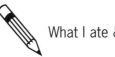 What I ate & drank, including alternatives

BREAKFAST
1 danish pastry or
Breakfast cake

NO SNACK

LUNCH
2 crispbreads with your
Choice of topping

NO SNACK

DINNER
On tea plate
2 lamb chops
2 vegetables—no potato
Gravy
Dessert of your choice

END OF DAY REWARD ☆
Small glass of wine or
1 frozen chocolate or
1 boiled sweet

WHAT DID YOU DRINK TODAY AND HOW MUCH? DID YOU EXERCISE?		
Tea and/or coffee?	Y / N	Amount:
Juice/sweetened/fizzy drinks?	Y / N	Amount:
Water?	Y / N	Amount:
Exercise?	Y / N	I did:

Time to start designing your own menu now. Keep to all the principles we have established. Why not get a recipe out of a low fat cooking book—you can be as adventurous as you feel. Just keep the food fresh, uncomplicated, NOT PROCESSED (if you are dying for a burger, then make your own) and keep the portion sizes down.

DAY 25 Thursday

BREAKFAST

SNACK

LUNCH

SNACK

DINNER
On tea plate

WHAT DID YOU DRINK TODAY AND HOW MUCH? DID YOU EXERCISE?		
Tea and/or coffee?	Y / N	Amount:
Juice/sweetened/fizzy drinks?	Y / N	Amount:
Water?	Y / N	Amount:
Exercise?	Y / N	I did:

DAY 26 Friday

BREAKFAST

SNACK

LUNCH

SNACK

DINNER
On tea plate

WHAT DID YOU DRINK TODAY AND HOW MUCH? DID YOU EXERCISE?		
Tea and/or coffee?	Y / N	Amount:
Juice/sweetened/fizzy drinks?	Y / N	Amount:
Water?	Y / N	Amount:
Exercise?	Y / N	I did:

DAY 27 Saturday

BREAKFAST

SNACK

LUNCH

SNACK

DINNER   ☆☆ + ☆
Weekly reward

WHAT DID YOU DRINK TODAY AND HOW MUCH? DID YOU EXERCISE?		
Tea and/or coffee?	Y / N	Amount:
Juice/sweetened/fizzy drinks?	Y / N	Amount:
Water?	Y / N	Amount:
Exercise?	Y / N	I did:

DAY 28 Sunday

BREAKFAST

SNACK

LUNCH
On tea plate—Sunday roast
Meat
3 vegetables +
1 small potato
Gravy
Dessert of your choice

NO SNACK

DINNER
On tea plate

DON'T FORGET TO FILL IN YOUR WEEKLY WEIGHTS AND MEASURES CHART.

HOW MUCH HAVE YOU LOST?

_____

TIME FOR YOUR BIG MONTH REWARD! WELL DONE.

DON'T STOP— KEEP GOING

DON'T STOP THOUGH—DO ANOTHER MONTH...

REALLY USEFUL INFORMATION

What vitamins do.

Vitamin	RDA	Benefits	Found in
Vitamin A	800ug	Good for eyesight, keeps skin healthy	Liver, eggs, butter, full fat milk, oily fish
Vitamin B6	2mg	Helps hormone production	Chicken, red meat, fish, bananas
Vitamin B12	1ug	Maintains healthy blood cells	Red meat, fish, breakfast cereal
Vitamin C	60mg	Maintains healthy immune system	Oranges, blackcurrants strawberries, kiwis
Vitamin D	5ug	Helps body absorb calcium	Eggs, cheese, oily fish
Folic Acid	200ug	Taken for first 12 weeks of pregnancy—help neural tube development	Breakfast cereal, spinach
Calcium	800mg	Essential for healthy teeth and bones	Milk, cheese, yoghurt, green beans, tofu
Iron	14mg	Essential for formation of red blood cells	Red meat, fish, eggs, baked beans, lentils
Zinc	15mg	Supports immune system	Red meat, sardines, cheese, nuts

WEBSITES WORTH A LOOK

Remember these sites change all the time so you might want to type words like diet, fitness, exercise, health etc. into your search engine and see what comes up. (correct as of 31/1/06)

www.bda.uk.com (latest food facts section)

www.ivillage.co.uk/dietandfitness

www.realage.com

www.sportengland.org

www.nutrition.org.uk

www.eatwell.gov.uk

www.bbc.co.uk/health

www.nutrition.gov (weight management section)

www.activeusa.com

www.besttreatments.co.uk

www.acefitness.org

www.americanheart.org

www.cdc.gov (Centers for Disease Control and Prevention)

www.who.int (World Health Organisation)

 # FURTHER READING

The Complete Guide to Sports Nutrition by Anita Bean, published by A&C Black

New Optimum Nutrition Bible by Patrick Holford, published by Piatkus Books

Essentials of Human Anatomy and Physiology by Elaine N. Marieb, published by Addison Wesley/Benjamin-Cummings

CROSSWORD ANSWERS

Across / Down answers (completed grid):

- 1 CARBOHYDRATE
- 2 B...
- 3 R...
- 4 FITNESS
- 5 E...
- 6 C...
- 7 M...
- 8 OIL
- 9 SALT
- 10 FAT
- 11 I...
- 12 Y...
- 13 V...
- 14 ENERGY
- 15 N...
- 16 N...
- 17 MUSCLES
- 18 T...
- 19 STEPS
- 20 DIET
- 21 BURN
- 22 W...
- 23 INGREDIENTS
- 24 KNOWLEDGE

```
C A R B O H Y D   R A T E
A     m         E
L   F I T N E S S     C m
O I L       A     T   F A
R     S A L T       F A T
I N   T         Y     A
E     R   V     O     B
S     E N E R G Y     N
  N   T   G     O     L
M U S C L E S     T   I
  T   H   T   S T E P S
  R       A   E     A m
D I E T   B U R N     W
  T       L   V       A
  I N G R E D I E N T S
  O           N       E
K N O W L E D G E     R
```

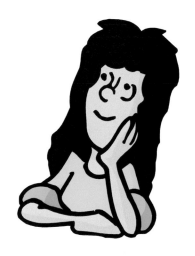

121

ACKNOWLEDGEMENTS

The author and publisher acknowledge the permission granted to reproduce the copyright material in this book. Every effort has been made to trace copyright holders and to obtain their permission for the use of copyright material. Where there are any errors or omissions in the above list, you should notify the publisher with any corrections that should be incorporated in future reprints or editions of this book.

Images were sourced from the following locations:
Clipart on pages 3, 36, 62 supplied by www.clipartheaven.com
Magnets on pages 14, 25, 38 are available for purchase from www.funkyfridge.com
Car image (photographer: Sencer Saygiver) on page 28, 32, 39 available on www.sxc.hu
Other images sourced from: Dreamtime, Stock Exchange, Randy Glasbergen & Fotolia

Book designed and typeset by Jodi-Lee Beder at The Elliott Partnership LLP.

The Elliott Partnership LLP.
556 Finchley Road
London, NW11 8DD
T: +44 (0)208 8201 8020
www.elliottpartnership.com

Printed by Nuffield Press Ltd.

Nuffield Press Ltd.
21 Nuffield Way
Abingdon
Oxon OX14 1RL

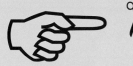

Please take a moment to fill in this form and return it to us.

GIVE US YOUR VIEWS

Name: ....

Address: ....

....

It would be greatly appreciated if you would fill in the feedback form to the right and return it to:

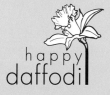

happy
daffodil

PO Box 57707

London

NW11 1BZ

E-mail: .... Age: .... Sex: Male ❑ Female ❑

How did you get hold of a copy of this book? ....

Was the book easy to follow?   Yes ❑ No ❑ ....

Can we contact you by post ❑ or E-mail ❑

Is there anything you would have liked to know that was not included in the book?

....

....

....

Would you be interested in the follow up book?   Yes ❑ No ❑

How much weight did you lose? ....

Do you have any hints and/or tips that you think other dieters would benefit from?

....

....

....

....

....

....

....

....

Please sign   Date

❑ You may use my hints and/or tips on your website or in further publications. [Please tick]

❑ I would like my name to appear alongside my hints and/or tips [Please tick]

(Where more than one person sends the same or similar tip, we will use the first name received.

Your name will appear like this: P.Smith Worcester

We will NOT pass on your details to any other party

THANK YOU.

Please send me:

£9.99 per copy includes packaging and 2nd class UK post.
Send me .... copy(ies)   £ ....

Continuation pack of: Exercise Plan, Short Term Goals
and Weights and Measurements forms to last you 2 months
@ £3.50 per pack. Send me .... pack(s)   £ ....

EXTRAS

Do you want recorded post? Add £0.99 per copy   £ ....

To post to Europe add £3.50 per copy   £ ....

To post to rest of world (excluding USA & Canada) add £6.50   £ ....

TOTAL £ ....

DETAILS

Full Name: ....

Address: ....

.... Postcode: ....

Daytime contact number: ....

WAYS TO BUY

Call 020 8201 8059
or Fax
020 8201 9020

www.itsnotrocketscience.info
for secure card payment

Make cheque payable to
'Happy Daffodil' and put your
name and address on back

Ask at your local book shop
quoting ISBN No:
0-9552911-0-0

TERMS AND CONDITIONS

1. Your order is sent securely packaged but, in the unlikely event that it arrives damaged, please call us immediately on 020 8201 8059 within 7 days of receipt.
2. Happy Daffodil will not be held liable for more than the actual amount paid per product.
3. PLEASE NOTE THAT IF THE SHRINK WRAPPED PLASTIC COVER HAS BEEN OPENED YOU WILL BE DEEMED TO HAVE ACCEPTED THE BOOK AND LOSE ANY RIGHT TO RETURN THE BOOK OR A REFUND. THIS DOES NOT LIMIT YOUR STATUTORY RIGHTS.

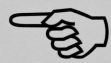

Do you need
continuation
sheets?

Do you know
someone who
would like
this book?
A great gift.

Why not buy
a copy for a
friend and
do the diet
together

Fill out the form to
the left and return
it to: ✉

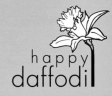
happy
daffodil

PO Box 57707

London

NW11 1BZ